# Lightning Strikes Twice

*Life After Two Brain Haemorrhages*

Tom East

# Benybont Books

https://www.benybont.org/
First published 2020
Copyright © Tom East, 2020

**ISBN 978-1-9162973-3-3**

*To Joseph, Edmund, Ping and Annabella*

## THANKS

I am so grateful for all the help and support I have been given in my two recoveries by so many people in a period of over twenty years. This includes medical and related staff, friends, former colleagues, neighbours and acquaintances. Also, I should not forget the many entire strangers who have shown me such uncondescending kindness. Most importantly, I must pay tribute to my immediate family, especially my dear wife Suki, who is no longer with us.

The naming convention I have followed is to use the first names of private individuals and (where I know them) both names of medical and other professionals of all kinds, providing I met them through their work. But I must emphasise that I owe a debt of gratitude to many people who are not named here.

# CONTENTS

## APPENDICES

# STROKES

Why is it that these devastating events are called 'strokes'? Although 'stroke' is one of those words with many meanings (at the stroke of one o'clock, a mark on something like a piece of paper or whiteboard, a particular style of swimming and so on) the first thing the hearer thinks of is a gentle, caressing touch. There is nothing gentle or caressing about a cerebrovascular accident or insult, to use the medical terms.

In fact, the use of the English word in the sense of 'apoplexy' dates back to the seventeenth century. It originally had connotations of the 'stroke of God's hand'. This may not go down well with those of us who are agnostic, but it is at least understandable. Pioneers of medicine like Hippocrates and Galen were familiar with the concept, knowing it as 'thunder-struck' or 'planet-struck'.

There are in fact two main kinds of medical stroke. Eighty-five percent occur when a person has a clot or other obstruction causing an interruption of the supply of blood to the brain. A smaller number (I belong to this category myself) suffer various kinds of bleeding in the brain's tissues. Either occurrence can cause damage, usually severe, often fatal.

If you want fancier terms, the first kind are called 'ischaemic strokes' and the latter 'haemorrhagic strokes'. Sometimes, a blockage to the blood supply can clear itself before any lasting damage is done. 'Episodes' (to use the unfortunate technical term) of this kind are called 'transient ischaemic attacks' or 'TIAs'. These are popularly, though not accurately, referred to as 'mini-strokes'.

You can get lost in these medical and etymological matters. If you've survived a stroke or someone close to you has, the primary questions that will be in your mind are 'what do I do now?' and 'how can life go on from here?' Although I've had two brain haemorrhages followed by two long periods of recovery, I wouldn't presume to think I can tell you the answers to these questions. Every stroke is different, in exactly the same way as every individual is different. The brain is hugely complex. Science doesn't pretend to know everything about it. I'm not even a scientist.

It would be pointless, not to say disrespectful, for me to attempt to lay down a series of homilies like 'you've got to keep fighting back', 'don't forget your sense of humour', 'accept that your life is going to change'. You'd, rightly, never forgive me if all I did was utter this sort of cliché. All I can do with honesty is to set down some of my experiences since March, 2000, in the hope someone may benefit from them, even if only slightly. This is my sole aim with this book.

The story is by no means all dark. If I have learned anything since the Millennium, it is how ready to be helpful, concerned, and considerate in a non-patronising way almost everyone has been. I have been given an object lesson in the finest qualities of human nature. It wasn't a lesson I sought and certainly not one I'd have had the courage to take if it had been offered to me, yet it is not one I can say I wholly regret.

The formal dedication to my family at the front of this book is richly deserved. No-one has helped me more than they. Yet I must also thank friends, other relatives, former colleagues, medical and other professionals of all kinds, acquaintances and even a large number of complete strangers, some of whose names I never found out, for the genuine kindness they have shown to me.

The only other thing I want to mention in this introduction is luck. My own experiences have been lucky ones. Some may prefer something more religious in tone; I prefer the neutral 'luck'.

It may sound odd to think of what happened to me on two occasions as 'lucky', especially when the doctors could find no reason why I should have had either haemorrhage in the first place. Yet everything could have been so much worse. I could have been struck down when one of my sons was sitting an important examination or when I was behind the wheel of a car.

The incidents themselves could have been worse. I could have, for example, been rendered immobile. I might have stepped off the planet altogether. I've been fortunate enough to make one reasonable recovery and am (I hope) still in the process of making a second. Yes, I've worked hard to repair my life but must acknowledge luck has been on my side.

I hope it's on the side of you or your beloved, too.

# Episode One
*Life Changes at the Millennium*

## [1] The Life Before

Not only did the year end at midnight on 31st December, 1999, but so did the old Millennium. As the new one arrived, the World didn't end, time didn't start to run backwards or do anything else peculiar and no aeroplanes fell out of the sky. The 'Millennium Bug' proved to have no bite. It turned out to be little more than mass hysteria on the part of people working in information technology. Firework displays were a different matter. Never before or since have I seen the skies lit up in quite the way they were as the clocks struck twelve.

My fifty-second birthday had been under two months before. Edmund, our elder son, had started the first year of his undergraduate course in the previous autumn. Joseph, his younger brother, was due to follow him, although to a different university, two years later. Neither Suki nor I had any significant problems in work and we both kept the minor ones in proportion, as I like to think we did all other aspects of our lives.

We hadn't taken our usual holiday abroad in 1999, but we'd had two enjoyable weeks in the United Kingdom. The first was by narrowboat on the Brecon and Monmouth Canal. Soon after this we travelled down to Penzance, hoping to see the total eclipse, the first visible from the British Isles since 1954. We'd booked to go on holiday to Madrid and Andalusia in the summer of 2000.

About ten years earlier, I'd resumed my interest in creative writing and so continued to satisfy the artistic impulses that have always been a feature of my life. These had suffered something of a long lapse in view of the many other things going on in the few decades before.

Roughly in chronological order, I moved from London to Wales, gained an external degree, married, started (belatedly, you might say) to build a career and did my bit in raising a family. Some of these things overlapped, naturally, but this order is about right. At the end of 1980 I received what I regard as my most important promotion in work then finished my degree only a few months before our first son was born.

As a family, our health at that time was good and the many things going together to build lives were at least satisfactory on all counts.

In short, we couldn't have had many legitimate complaints about the way things were progressing.

Unlike the one we were to experience a year later; I remember the winter of 1999/2000 as mild and uneventful. Indeed, I recall reading a newspaper column confidently but prematurely informing us that snow had now become a thing of the past. At all events, we were certainly enjoying the early spring and looking forward to the summer ahead. The only other piece of news I recall from that time was when Dr Harold Shipman shook the faith of people in the medical profession by being convicted of his alarming crimes. He was the only British doctor to be found guilty of murdering patients on such a horrific scale.

All I remember from work in the period immediately before I all at once and unexpectedly became an employee no more was attending a pensions meeting in Cardiff on Monday 20th March, 2000. I have no clue as to what subjects were up for discussion but, if these included anything on ill-health retirement, it would have been an extreme irony. In not much more than 36 hours I would be taking the first step to becoming eligible for a pension myself.

## [2] And Then it Went Dark

Tuesday, 21st March, 2000 started like any other working day. I don't remember anything special about it, weather-, work- or otherwise. The day before, I'd been to Cardiff for a pensions meeting but I'm sure I didn't go far for any work reason on the Tuesday.

More than likely I did nothing more than go for a stroll at lunchtime. This was usually a duller experience in my hometown than it had been when I'd worked in Cardiff four years earlier, but I still appreciated the opportunity to blow some of the morning's dust away. Rarely did I not take the chance to leave the office for at least twenty minutes, even on those days when the weather was poor, and I was busy.

I do remember the meal I had at home that evening. It was a baked potato with mince; simple fare but something I liked. At around 8:30pm, I drove Suki to work. She was at that time a nurse in the local hospital working part-time, two nights a week.

When I reached home, I wanted to arrange to call on a friend and near-neighbour of mine, Joyce. I was playing postman for the editor of a local small press magazine, Arthur, and had a few copies of his magazine, *Cambrensis*, to deliver. At the time, Joyce was chairman of our local writers' group and I was the treasurer. So, after we'd eaten, I telephoned, and she told me it would be fine for me to call. The magazines were quickly dealt with and we then had a brief chat. I don't remember the details of our conversation, but it was hardly likely to have been of any great moment, even at the level of the business of the writers' circle, which was flourishing at the time.

But the events of around 9pm will be forever burned into my memory. At least, the events before I lost consciousness will be.

Joyce had left the room for a moment. As she returned, I glanced up from the chair on which I was sitting. There was nothing unusual or sudden in my movement. When I looked up,

I felt a warm, though couldn't honestly say unpleasant, gentle squirting sensation, quite literally inside my head. This may sound a strange thing, but I am clear this was the case: I noted it carefully at the time and now remember it only too well. I remarked something about 'feeling funny', adding that I was developing a headache (this had always been a rare event for me). Then I tried to get up and half-slid to the floor. Joyce helped me back to my seat in the chair.

I then knew a stretching, pins-and-needles, feeling in the muscles at the side of my face. It wasn't possible to locate exactly where on my face the problem was. The whole thing felt wrong to me.

'Can I have a mirror?' I asked Joyce.

'A mirror?' She tried to laugh but I could see her expression was becoming concerned. 'Now you're becoming vain.'

'Go home to Joseph,' I said, with some difficulty. I meant that I wanted to go to my younger son, who I knew was at home at the time.

'You're not going anywhere,' Joyce said. 'I'm getting a doctor.'

'Ring Joseph,' I said.

She did. Our homes are only fifty or sixty yards apart and he'd arrived within minutes. Joyce went to bring him in. She'd left the front door ajar, but Joseph had gone to the back door. She walked around the side of her house.

While she was doing this, I rose and stumbled over to the mirror on her sideboard to see what was wrong with my face. I could make out some distortion in my features, although only for a second or two. This was because I couldn't maintain my balance, even with the support of the sideboard. I fell backwards. When Joyce and Joseph came into the room moments later, I was sprawled on the floor, being sick. I was too heavy to be lifted back onto the chair, so they tried to make me comfortable where

I was. Joyce telephoned for an ambulance and made a call to Suki, who was working at the hospital to where I'd soon be heading.

Joyce wiped my face with a wet flannel and covered me with a blanket. She gave me a pillow for support as I lay there, waiting for the ambulance. The phone rang a couple of times as I waited but I had my eyes closed. I wasn't taking much notice of the brief conversations I could hear around me or my surroundings, even though I was still conscious.

I'm not sure how long it took for the paramedics to arrive, although I had the impression this wasn't many minutes. But my perceptions were unreliable by that stage. I know all the time I was lying on the floor, no more than half-conscious of what was going on around me. At the same time, I was somehow becoming vaguely and miserably aware of what must have happened.

When they arrived, the crew efficiently eased me onto a stretcher, and carried their burden to the ambulance. Joseph ran home to lock up our house.

Perhaps wrongly, I remember the vehicle as being parked on the other side of the road. All the time the paramedics were working, I was trying to carry on a conversation with one of them. I don't know if he could understand anything of what I was saying, although I have to doubt it. He was telling me to calm down and rest.

Then it went dark.

# [3] Inpatient

My memory is blank for the first three days after I lost consciousness in the ambulance and sparse for the next week. From my own recollections, therefore, I am unable to put together a full, or even reasonably complete, account of my time in the Casualty or Medical Assessment Units, nor the short time I spent in the main ward before being transferred to a side ward, nor indeed of my first few days in that side ward.

Apparently, though, I was conscious for a lot of this time and even tried to take part in a few conversations. On 22nd March, the day after I was admitted to hospital, several members of my family were 'gathered around my bedside' in traditional fashion. I'm told that from time to time I made mumbled contributions to proceedings, sometimes with eyes closed and sometimes with eyes open.

Joyce, the woman who was the main witness to my first 'episode', tells me she called into the hospital on that same day and again on 23rd. On the second occasion I opened my eyes and asked her, 'who brought you?' She was recovering from a cataract operation and at the time couldn't have driven herself. Somehow, I must have reasoned this. My then boss in work came to see me around the same time. He later told me I opened my eyes briefly and said, 'Don't worry, Allan.'

I have no recollection of any of these three occasions, but accounts of all of them have been given to me more than once by the people concerned and I have no reason to doubt their veracity.

In the second part of April, 2000, not long after I'd been discharged, my wife Suki helped me to put together a 'diary of events' for my three weeks in hospital. This has been reproduced as appendix one (page 143) for the sake of completeness in this record. In this section, therefore, I feel free to concentrate on memories I can claim as my own.

But, first of all, I should record that Suki was there for the greater part of each day and for most nights of my three-week stay. On the two nights she wasn't, one or other of my sons slept near to my hospital bed. Not only that, but Suki was on sick leave throughout the three weeks and became my de facto nurse on a one-to-one basis. The regular staff on the ward did most of the 'professional' things, like administering drugs, and naturally they talked to me, but Suki provided all the one-to-one bedside care like bathing and washing. So, I had the best possible nursing attention! I am so grateful for it.

The first real memory I have that is more than a fragment is from 2nd April, 2000. My sons were both with me at the time. I wandered from the side ward into the main ward and, as Edmund and Joseph described it, started to 'interview' some of the patients. I don't recall the detail of these 'interviews', although do remember the alarmed expressions of the patients.

The next occasion I remember – it may even have been on the same day - is doing some exercises under the instruction of the physiotherapist, Siân, whilst hanging on for grim life to the bed. Apparently, I'd got out of bed for the first time the day before and then performed similar exercises for her. I'd even done a few stretches before this whilst I was still confined to bed. I have no memory of any of these things. What I do remember very clearly is a day, almost a week later, when Siân called in to see me. I was alone in the side room, sitting in the chair.

'Why aren't you dressed?' she said. I was wearing a dressing gown.

I mumbled something.

'Well, I know *I'd* want to get dressed properly.'

From that time until my discharge some days later, I ensured I was dressed whenever I was out of bed.

By that time, I was walking down to the physiotherapists' room for most of my exercise sessions, or going for quite long walks around the hospital, with Edmund and Joseph on either side. I felt immense pride at being able (with help!) to ascend and descend the short flight of steps linking the upstairs floor, where the wards were sited, with the lower floor and main corridor. Together with Suki, on one occasion we went to the hospital canteen. It was hardly a five-star dining experience, but it made a wonderful change to eat away from the ward.

One day not long after I'd got out of bed for the first time, stands out vividly in my mind. I'd wanted a 'proper' bath (presumably after the 'bed baths' of which I have no memory). Suki helped me into the shower-room. At least, I call it a shower room, although in my memory is of nothing more than the hose affair (presumably Suki had taken down the shower hose) used to wash me. I couldn't stand up, so sat or knelt on the floor while Suki 'hosed' and soaped me.

She wanted me to change my position slightly, by unfolding my leg from beneath me. I simply couldn't do it and started to laugh uncontrollably at the sheer silliness of the situation. Suki couldn't help but join in the laughter with me. Eventually, when I regained control of myself, we both made a supreme effort to get my leg in the required position and finally were able to complete the task. Drying with the white hospital towel felt superb. I was clean again. I felt I was washing away my 'imprisonment' in a hospital bed.

As the days went on and I continued my gradual recovery, I began to feel intolerant of daily routine in the ward. On 9th and 10th April, with exhausting effort, I wrote some strange notes and drew some weird sketches on hospital notepaper. These have survived and I reproduce them as appendices two and three (pages 145 and 147). If you can't make out what all of them are supposed to represent, you're not the only one. Neither can I.

There is one note I made on 10th April that will be intelligible to most who read it. In peculiar but clear handwriting I've written 'I'm bored!' By this time, Suki was campaigning on my behalf for my discharge. On Tuesday, 11th April I was watching the consultant, Dr Helen Parry making her round of the ward, and slowly getting nearer to me. Suki had told me that the consultant *might* discharge me on that day, but not to get my hopes up too high. It seemed Dr Parry wanted me to remain as an in-patient until the end of the month and would have insisted on it were Suki not a qualified nurse. I was overjoyed when the doctor at last reached my side ward and told me I could go.

Without delay, Suki telephoned our friend Breda. She'd been good enough to say she'd give us both a lift home. We quickly packed and waited for her in the reception area at the front of the hospital. Seeing her car drive past the entrance was like seeing the arrival of the scriptural wingéd chariot. Only this one would be taking me back to the land of the living, not away from it.

# The Long Road Back

# [4] Out of Hospital

I'd been discharged from the hospital. I was free! But I must admit to much trepidation when I started properly to realise I'd have to cope with a world I knew would now be strange and new to me as I watched Breda's car being parked.

Breda has a few health problems of her own but loves to drive and is unfailingly cheerful. Both of us were glad to see her car driving into the car park. Suki had spent most of her time over the last three weeks in the hospital and I'd been there for the whole of this time. It certainly did feel like I was making my escape.

Soon after finding myself at home, Suki told me I should telephone Joyce to let her know I was out of hospital. She knew Joyce had been staying with her friend in Warwickshire but was due back that same day.

Neither of us was aware of this then but, a short time before, Joyce had telephoned our house and, when she could get no reply, she rang the hospital. The staff told her I'd been discharged an hour before. My phone call came almost immediately after they told her this. Joyce has furnished me with this transcription of our conversation:

R: *Hello?*
J: *[Speechless with surprise]*
R: *Sorry; wrong number.*
J: *No. No. It is me. I can't believe it's you.*
R: *[Laughs]*
J: *How are you?*
R: *A bit bothered and bewildered.*
J: *I'd have trouble saying that.*

The next morning, Joyce visited. I was sitting in a chair, wearing a dressing gown. She told me I was looking well. I'm not sure I was feeling altogether well at this stage, but I knew I was glad to be sitting in the chair at home rather than the one next to my hospital bed.

On the Friday evening of the same week, our friends Ewart and Brenda took us out for a short drive. I remember the cars flashing past on the road and not being able to focus on them, or on our surroundings. It was if I were a slow-motion being in a high-speed world. I wondered whether I'd ever be able to drive again for myself and had to acknowledge being a long way from normality that stage. Leaving aside the short return journey from the hospital, this was my first venture into the outside world. I relished it, despite my disorientation. I delighted in it when we stopped at a pub on the way home and I was able to enjoy my first pint in the best part of a month.

It wasn't all to be plain sailing. The day after my pub visit, Saturday, 15th April, saw me sitting down at the table at home to have a largish roast meal with the family. Part of the way through, I knew I couldn't continue. I had to get up from the table and go upstairs for a rest.

Whilst lying on the bed, no more than half-dozing, I had the most unusual experience. I have vivid memories of it, though am not sure I can describe it in a way that would be meaningful to anyone else. I heard the sound of an aeroplane flying above. Notes I made later that same afternoon (and which I've refrained from editing) read:

*Aeroplane:*
*Just me and it in the Universe*
*Hear noise of (beforehand)*
*Mystic connection with pilot + passengers. There and here.*
*Slight delirium of pre-sleep*
*Humming noise*

These notes might not be very explicatory, but they do at least have the advantage of being current. What happened was that I seemed to be in two places at the same time. One of 'me' was still lying on the bed, whilst 'the other' was standing up inside the cabin of the aeroplane – not a large one, as I recall from its sound. I was looking down at the seated passengers. For some reason there was a small cable stretched above me on the top of the passenger compartment. This was exactly like those there used to be on London buses many years ago, right down to the same off-white of the cable used to sound the 'start/stop' bell of the bus.

The others on the aeroplane were looking up toward at me. Although nobody said anything, they seemed slightly – no more than slightly – surprised to see me standing there. I didn't look over my shoulder but was somehow aware that the pilot was seated behind me at the controls with his door open. Although he was also saying nothing, I knew he wanted me to sit down.

Gradually, the 'me' on the bed became the dominant one and lost touch with 'the other'. For some time afterwards, long after the sound of the aeroplane should have been audible, I continued to hear a humming sound. Eventually, I fell asleep and felt quite refreshed when I awoke.

It was a most peculiar experience. I'm certainly not going to try to put forward any rational explanation for it, although of course my brain could hardly be described as functioning normally at the time. There was certainly an aeroplane passing above. I had heard it approaching. My haemorrhage had been under a month before and, at that time, my dosage of medication was four times what it was soon after to become.

As best I could, I tried to resume my normal life. This wasn't easy. For the first few days I couldn't remember simple things, like how to log in to my computer. My sons had to show me how to do it. My double-vision prevented me from watching much television: the only thing I could do it at this stage was to cover up one eye by means of a handkerchief stuffed behind one lens of my spectacles. Even listening to the radio made me tired after no more than twenty minutes. I read, and even wrote, a few fragmentary pieces but was unable to read a whole book until the middle of May.

Still, I tried to do what I could. My sons, one on each side of me when they were both around, took me for walks. These had to be of fairly short distance for the first week or so but soon increased in length and, before too much longer, I was pleased to find I no longer needed support.

I was taking my first faltering steps on the long road to recovery.

## [5] Around Carreg Cennan

In the middle of March, 2000, only a week or so before my life was to change so drastically, Suki and I had discussed visiting the castle of Carreg Cennan with our friends, Ewart and Brenda. They'd made it their practice to take a walk around the castle over the Christmas and New Year holiday. Our friends were always ecstatic about the castle's dramatic setting atop a rock in the Carmarthenshire countryside, not far from the famously named village of Bethlehem. 'Carreg' does indeed mean 'stone' or 'rock', whilst 'Cennan' or 'Cennen', is derived from the name of the small brook to the south of the castle, Afon Cennen.

Over the final Christmas of the old Millennium, Ewart and Brenda hadn't managed to find time for their usual walk but, such was the glorious picture they'd painted, we were immediately sold on the idea of joining them for a delayed ramble. Easter was late that year; in fact, it fell on the latest dates it had during my whole lifetime up to that point. We agreed in mid-March the holiday weekend would be the ideal time to make the journey.

But the world can change in an instant. I was to find myself in hospital as the date for the venture was drawing near. Although I was to be discharged early, by that time mid-April was almost upon us and the scheduled date for our walk was under two weeks away. Our plan looked like it would become nothing more than a pious intention.

But, as the days passed, I made good progress. Ewart and Brenda took us out to a few nearby places for gentle drives. As the Easter weekend arrived, I persuaded them to take us to Carreg Cennan as we'd originally proposed. After all, my argument went, we could always limit ourselves to a cup of coffee and a look out of the large glass windows in the café they'd told us about, even if I wasn't up to making more than a short walk.

The walking shoes I'd insisted on wearing 'just in case' may have told a different story.

We enjoyed glorious weather for our day out. When we reached the car park, I discussed with Ewart the possibility of doing part of the walk around the castle. So, we approached the starting point for the walk instead going to the coffee-shop. The next part I remember very clearly: the image of the direction signs is lucid in my mind to this day. There was a choice of routes. One sign pointed to the west and read 'one-and-a-half miles', the other to the east and read 'four-and-a-half miles'. My three companions gave me choice of which to follow for a short distance.

After only a brief hesitation, I said we should follow the longer path to the east. It is hard now for me to reconstruct my thought processes so many years later but I know I briefly (and somewhat illogically; I know) considered the 'family walks' book I had published a mere seven years before. The route might have been moderately long, even if I knew the terrain wasn't especially demanding. On the other hand, I had been discharged from hospital less than a fortnight before. I remembered the consultant's original view that I should still at this date be in my hospital bed. Would I be pushing my luck? Sheer bloody-mindedness on my part led us to the east. Whatever the other three were thinking, I had no intention of going only part way along the path.

We set out and, while we were still heading eastwards through the wooded Cennen Valley, I began to regret my decision. My legs were starting to ache. I was very conscious about feeling an acute lack of strength in my body as The Black Mountain, or Picws Du, the westernmost edge of The Beacons ranges, came into view. By the time we'd crossed our second stile before reaching Hengrofft Farm, I'd already needed three lengthy halts simply to draw breath.

After the farm there was some compensation in the shape of what were to be perhaps the most impressive views of the castle above us. Its legendary association with an earlier fortress built by Sir Urien, one of King Arthur's knights, probably is no more than legendary, but, looking upward from this point, it is easy to believe otherwise.

Further to the south some prehistoric stone cairns were visible on the skyline. Ewart tried to draw my attention to these but, to be honest, by this stage I was too tired to do much more than put my head down and keep walking. The usual pleasures of country rambles had to make way for the endurance test this one had quickly become.

After what seemed an age, we at last found ourselves approaching the end of the walk. One of the final stretches was a steep section (it seemed almost vertical to me) following a challenging succession of three stiles. By this time, my legs were weak and wobbly. I needed physical help to get over the last two stiles.

Finally, the car park came into view once more. We'd taken over four hours to follow a route that should have been covered with no difficulty in two-and-a-half hours, but we'd made it. I was very tired but hugely proud, even if I couldn't muster the strength to express my feelings. The full hour we spent in the coffee shop was well-deserved, so it seemed to me. Anyway, I couldn't have summoned the energy to have left much before this.

*

A few weeks later, the four of us made a less demanding walk along the broad ridge between the Ogmore and Garw Valleys. Before too much longer, we were once again making frequent excursions to places like the 'Waterfall Country' above the Vale of Neath, the flat sands of our nearest beach of Merthyr Mawr and the splendid dunes backing them.

A few years afterwards, Suki and I made the nine-mile walking round trip from Welwyn in Hertfordshire to 'Shaw's Corner' in Ayot St Lawrence. It was a blazing hot day and we'd soon consumed all the water in the four large bottles we'd brought with us. We needed to supplement our hydration by stopping in a couple of pubs along the way. It didn't seem to matter that we found the cottage closed on our arrival. We had the garden to ourselves, just as George Bernard Shaw would have done in the summers from 1906 until his death in 1950.

With Ewart and Brenda, we climbed Pen-y-fan and the adjacent peak of Corn Du. At 2907 feet, the former is the highest peak in Britain south of Cadair Idris. This might not be quite as impressive as it sounds; the ascent from Storey Arms on the A470 is undemanding. My younger son, Joseph, made it when he was six.

The descent with my double vision was a far sterner challenge. Perhaps I should maintain my dignity and simply tell you that I relied heavily on the walking staff I carried to feel my way ahead and act as a brake. But I won't. Instead I'll be honest and tell you I managed to slither gracefully over onto my backside three times as we made the return journey.

*

In February, 2015, almost fifteen years after my first walk around Carreg Cennan, the four of us made another visit. This time, we merely drank a cup of coffee and looked out of the window of the café!

## [6] Two Games of Cricket

Before I went into hospital, I'd booked tickets for a day of the first home cricket Test Match of the season for the four of us – Suki, Edmund, Joseph and me. This was to be against Zimbabwe, still then a Test nation.

The day we'd chosen was Saturday, 20th May, 2000. This wasn't much more than a month after my discharge from hospital, but I decided to make the trek to Lords Cricket Ground regardless. Zimbabwe was by then beginning to fall apart as a cricketing nation as well as in other ways, but I'd never seen them. And there was the matter of the not insignificant cost of the tickets.

In the event Joseph, couldn't come with us. He was in his first 'A'-level year and had recently started a Saturday job. Already he was planning for his years in university to come. His elder brother, Edmund, was in his first university year. Soon after my hospital discharge, I'd been pleased to be able to assure them both that their higher education plans would not be disrupted by my dramatically changed circumstances.

On the train to London, I began to wonder if I'd made the right decision in coming to London at all. Because of my double vision, still then at its most severe, it was difficult for me to read. For the same reason, it wasn't much fun to look out of the window. The fields, hedges and buildings whipped by with bewildering rapidity before I could begin to focus on them. And my speech difficulties meant I couldn't be much of a conversationalist.

I was used to travelling to the capital by train, but this seemed the longest rail journey I'd made in my life. My doubts were compounded on the tube journey from Paddington to St John's Wood. The press of people in the crowded underground carriage wasn't easy for me to cope with. It was something I'd hardly noticed in the past.

Rather than anticipating any pleasures to come, I knew simple relief when we found our seats in the stand.

The match itself was undistinguished. I recall that Mike Atherton, Darren Gough and Andrew Flintoff played for England. Andy Flower, later to have mixed fortunes as the England coach, was one of the Zimbabwe players. I remember little else. Zimbabwe was batting and proved to be extremely fragile. The team's wickets fell at regular intervals and an easy victory for England was announced next day, after we'd gone home.

My greatest preoccupations were not with the cricket. It wasn't the brightest of May days and often I found it to be downright cold. I was grateful for the blanket Suki had insisted I bring along. I found it difficult to focus my eyes on the bowling and batting. Which of the two images I could see should I concentrate on? Looking back upon it, the day wasn't entirely wasted: I'd done some useful eyesight training that would help me in the years to come.

After another long train journey (it didn't seem as long as the outward journey because I dozed part of the way) we at last arrived at home at a fairly late hour. I was shattered. But at least I'd made it.

*

During the nineteen-nineties, we as a family had been regular cricket-goers. When our County side, Glamorgan, switched to an imaginative pricing policy, we were pleased to count ourselves among its rapidly increasing membership. The four of us used our season tickets to attend most of the home Sunday one-day matches and quite a number of single days of the County Championship matches.

We also regularly attended one Test Match a year, went along with pleasure whenever our County hosted an overseas Test side and attended a few other international matches. I well remember seeing New Zealand overcoming the odds to beat Australia in a 1999 World Cup match held in Cardiff. Don't tell my brother-in-law Phil from Western Australia, but the four of us became honorary New Zealanders on that day.

A few months after the Zimbabwe Test Match, a friend did take me to Swansea where Glamorgan were playing in the County Championship, but it seemed to me that my days of enjoying cricket matches were to be a thing of the past. Fortunately, this was to change on 23rd June, 2012.

The week before, on Father's Day, my sons had surprised me. They'd bought tickets for the three of us to attend the representative one-day match between Wales and England to be held at Cardiff. It didn't have Test Match status; the rivalry was more intense than that of a mere Test Match.

England had its Test team on display. Its members were no doubt expecting a comfortable warm-up, a gentle tuning for the summer ahead; the Wales' side largely comprised Glamorgan players. There were, though, some interesting additions, like the exceptionally talented South African all-rounder, Jacques Kallis. I'd like to have understood the convoluted logic qualifying him for the Wales' side. He'd been Glamorgan's overseas player three years before, but Kallis was most definitely South African born and bred.

England batted first and achieved a miserably low score. None of the batsmen shone. For Glamorgan, Robert Croft and Darren Thomas took two wickets apiece. There were some inglorious runs-out, adding to England's misery. Kallis claimed only one wicket, so couldn't be said to have been the architect of England's downfall.

When it was England's turn to bowl, the match really came to life. The sun shone and the beer flowed through the crowd. This was what cricket was all about. The highlight for me, as for most of the crowd, was Matthew Hoggard's bowling. Hoggard was at that time tipped to be England's star bowler but had an unfortunate tendency to bowl wide. In what was surely one of the classics of sledging, every time he ran up to bowl, the crowd chanted:

*'Hoggie! Hoggie! Hoggie! Wide! Wide! Wide!'*

Hoggard duly obliged by bowling more wides and no-balls than usual. The crowd certainly played on his nerves. You had to feel almost sorry for him. Almost, that is. Another bowler who received more than his share of barracking from the crowd was Ronnie Irani. At the time he was being promoted as England's saviour in one day cricket. His stock fell after that day.

The match ended in a massive win for Wales. Steve James had a large not-out score as the game finished. Batting with him was Jacques Kallis, who had only just come in and started to collect runs. Like his bowling, his batting, though as competent as usual, was by no means the key factor in the result. The highly partisan crowd went home happy in the sun.

No-one was happier than me. I was enjoying cricket again.

## [7] Well-Wishers

A thing greatly lifting my spirits during the few months after my discharge from hospital was the large number of contacts I received from people who wanted to wish me well. These came by way of letter, 'get well card' and personal visit: at that time, fewer people used e-mail or the welter of electronic means of communication now available to us now. Needless to say, all were welcome and I'm sure each one did me a power of good. The callers were from across South Wales and beyond.

It would be wrong of me to try to name or even describe the actions of too many individuals. I might omit someone. This would be unforgivable. However, I would like to mention my old friend Dave, whom I have known for well over sixty years. He travelled from Surrey to see me soon after I was out of hospital. At that time, I could hardly talk, but the image of myself staring dumbly at our mantelpiece is forever burned into my mind.

I did manage to reply to all of the letters, although it was getting into summer before I felt up to doing this. What I've done is reproduce one of those letters sent in reply (made anonymous, naturally) as appendix five, page 151. I'm not trying to say that this letter is representative in any way – I hope my letters were too individual for that – but it does give some insight into the way I felt, five months after my first haemorrhage.

Reading this letter now, there is no denying that I was trying to put a positive spin on events. It had been quite clear to me for some time that I wouldn't be returning to work. My dexterity still had a long way to go. My double vision was more than 'occasional' – it was accentuated in a spectacular way every time I was mobile, even though I was beginning to learn by then how to cope with this problem.

Hardest for me to endure was the fact that my speech was characterised by rather more than a 'slight impediment'. The upbeat tone came partly, I believe, from the letter to my would-be holiday insurers, from which I quoted. In the event, the letter to the insurance company didn't have the hoped-for result. In true 'computer says no' tradition, they refused to give me any kind of cover. The consequences of this I've described in section 9, page 47.

Yet the letter I put together was far from being a complete work of fiction. I was indeed making a rapid recovery at that stage. I had made the longish walks described. My medication had been halved from the original prescription and was soon to be halved again.

My speech *was* progressing well, if more slowly than everything else, by that stage. The rate of improvement for this slowed considerably around the time I wrote those optimistic words. Still, as the letter to my well-wisher puts it (in a slightly different context) 'But *c'est la vie*, and taking everything into account I was extremely lucky.'

## [8] The Eyes Have It

Since 21st March, 2000 I have suffered from diplopia, or double vision. This is something to which you never wholly become accustomed, although you can, with effort, get used to living with it and making the numerous adjustments daily life requires. For all the years since, there has been no significant easing (or worsening) in my degree of double vision; although obviously immediately after the times of my crises there have been other things I've had find a way to handle along with it. These were tough in the early days. I've long since given up expecting there to be any real change to my diplopia.

All humans with binocular vision – nearly all of us – have two slightly different images channelled to our brains. This is what you'd assume to be the case if you think about it. Our eyes are sited some inches apart and so see slightly different images. The closer the object viewed, the more different the images will be. In most cases, our brains do the necessary matching up of the images to ensure we see one stereoscopic object and not two overlapping pictures.

One of the most complex things our enormously sophisticated brains do is to convert the light absorbed by the photoreceptor cells in our retinas to the images we actually see. These images give us information on contrast, colour, motion, and many other things in the world about us. The problem of converting light into something we can visually understand in such ways is far beyond the capabilities of any computer on Earth at present. Vision is truly a partnership between brain and eye. It is an impressive one.

In 2000, the neural pathways and the process for the matching of images in my own brain were damaged. Apart from myopia (short sightedness), which was diagnosed when I was twelve and was readily corrected by spectacles, my eyes themselves are fine, apart from what I mention in the last section, page 137.

It is my brain that has the difficulty. Specifically, the stereoscopic matching in my case is far less than perfect. If the object is close by, or if I have to look upwards or (especially) downwards to see it, the two images may not even overlap. They can be in different places, no more than proximate to each other. This can make simple tasks like, for example, descending a flight of stairs or reading a printed page something of a challenge. Even simple tasks like eating a meal off a plate before me need careful concentration, otherwise I may attempt to slice up the tablecloth.

Closing one eye when coming down a staircase or steps removes the double vision, obviously, but it also removes all sense of depth. I have no clue as to whether I'm coming down a few inches or a few feet. This can be a disconcerting experience in an unfamiliar place. Stepping down gingerly from a height which in the event proves to be only an inch-and-a-half can be almost as bad as getting a jolt from an unexpected descent of eighteen inches. Going up a flight of stairs is far easier because the contrast between light and shadow gives sufficient visual clues to the shape and depth of the step, even with one eye closed.

Naturally, not all descents can be down regular steps. Some walking has to be done over terrain which amounts to inclines and descents as, for example, when going over stony, rough ground. Even in urban spaces sudden raising or lowering of the ground is not rare. This is a thing always demanding alertness to the environment. All of these lessons, and more, I was to learn the hard way.

In the summer of the year 2000, after my first haemorrhage, I didn't understand all that this meant. I was making rapid progress with most aspects of my recovery. Even my speech did seem to be improving, although the rate of progress in this was to slow right down after a few months. I thought my visual difficulties would fit somewhere into this general pattern and the problem would be only temporary. The one question in my mind in the first half of the year was whether 'temporary' was to mean short- or long-term.

When my last connection with our local hospital became the one with the orthoptist, Lorraine Floyd, I still retained this optimism, even though with a growing realisation that the difficulties were clearly not to be short-lived. I even took some pride at being able and happy to walk the three or so miles for my appointments with her. At these she tried a variety of stick-on prismatic lenses with my spectacles. The success of the prisms was limited. They helped to some degree when I could keep my head still, as when trying to read the letters on a standard sight-test chart, but they were of no use at all when I had to move my head. This, of course, is what we have to do in normal living. It's why we have a neck.

I continued to attend the appointments with Lorraine for most or all of the year. She would make conscientious tests and measures but there was little to give me any practical help. When she went on maternity leave she suggested that, whilst there might not be a great deal of practical benefit for me to see her replacement, I might like to come and see her again when she returned to duty later in 2001. There didn't seem to me to be any point in doing this, so I let it lapse.

Meanwhile, I was finding ways to cope. I read my first novel in May, 2000 by the process of stuffing a handkerchief behind the left-hand lens of my reading spectacles. Later, I covered the lens with sticking plaster. This was effective, if unsightly and messy. When mobile, especially when going upwards or downwards, I took extreme care and didn't hesitate to close one eye when I needed to.

I learned to count items of food with one eye closed – something which I found to be advisable to do frequently. It can be disappointing to think you have three or four sausages on a plate and then find you have only two. Mirages don't have quite the same flavour! If I wanted to pick up a small object, I found it paid to close one eye to prevent myself grabbing at empty space. I am not being flippant here: these are matters I have to think about all the time.

Small compensations are continually necessary. For no good, reason, one early experience has stayed with me particularly. I was on a bus journey to my home. The nearest push-button to ring the bell in order to stop the bus was at the back of the seat opposite my own. My problem was that a woman passenger was sitting in a relaxed position with her head a few inches from the bell-push. Normally, the natural thing to do would have been to lean over slightly to press the button. But I knew that, in my case, I might miss the button and press the back of her head instead. The consequences might have been interesting, to say the least.

The alternative would have been for me to stand up and push the button sited two rows ahead. I spent some time debating with myself which option to choose. I was relieved when she dismounted two bus stops before me. But then, at the next stop another passenger took the seat. In the end I took the decision to press the button nearest me, concentrating ridiculously hard to ensure my aim was true and I did not cause an incident.

All of these things I have now come to accept as a required part of living. I am conscious that the adjustments I have constantly to make slow me down. On occasion it may seem to others that I have more disabilities than I actually do. Never mind; it is all part of the survival process. When I can walk on the flat I do it at an averagely fast speed and can do so for long distances. Unless they know or speak to me, people would have no reason to think I have a problem. Suki even told me I looked well when I was in hospital for the second time in 2010.

Following the cessation of my appointments with the orthoptist, I have nothing more than routine sight tests with my optician. These are annual in my case. They have been at that frequency for around 25 years. The reason for this was that my mother had glaucoma (controlled) and had nothing to do with my own neural problems. The optometrist knew about these, naturally, but nothing additional beyond the normal visual check on the physical health of my eyes was necessary.

Earlier in this century, on one of my annual sight tests, I decided to ask if I could have reading glasses in which the left-hand lens was made from clouded material. It seemed a reasonable idea to me; it would look neater than sticking tape and it seemed better not to waste an optical lens. The optician told me this could be done but seemed surprised.

'You must get this request all the time,' I said.

'No; not really,' she replied. 'In fact, you're the first to ask.'

## [9] Uninsured Spain

In February or March, 2000, I believe it was, but at any rate before my haemorrhage, we'd booked a holiday to go in early September to Madrid and Andalusia. We hadn't bought an insurance policy, intending to get one later in the year.

This put me in a quandary. With less than six months between my health spectacular and the departure date for Spain, no-one would insure me, even at an overblown premium. Over the summer, Suki and I talked about the problem. The outcome, and I really did think long and hard about it, was that I decided to travel uninsured. Mine was a personal decision: I am not recommending it as a course of action for anyone else to follow.

We'd paid a significant deposit on the holiday which we'd forfeit, but this wasn't the main consideration. After a few visits to various parts of the north of the country, Southern Spain was a part of the world I'd long wanted to visit, and the greater part of my recovery was proceeding apace. The deciding factor was that I resented what I unreasonably felt to be my entrapment.

The flight and our visits to the cities of Madrid and Toledo went smoothly, without incident. Then we travelled by coach to Cordoba, which was to be our base in the south. On the way we stopped at a group of windmills, portrayed as 'Don Quixote's Windmills.' They were indeed of the round tower type I'd seen in illustrations accompanying short popular extracts from the long novel. It didn't seem to matter that Quixote was a fictional creation by Miguel de Cervantes Saavedra rather than a character from history. I've heard the guides on Thames Cruisers pointing out, in a similar straight-faced way, the area of London where Bill Sikes met his end.

I felt rather like some sort of Don Quixote figure myself as I ascended the quite small slopes leading to the windmills. What should I do once I'd climbed their dizzying peaks? I don't remember what we actually did. I probably took some photographs on my old-style SLR camera. The digital revolution in photography was only just beginning to get into its stride at that time and, like most people then, I relied on chemical prints or transparencies

It was to be the following Christmas before I had my first digital camera. If I'd carried it with me on that day, no doubt I'd have used it freely. I'm entirely sure the resulting pictures would have long disappeared into cyberspace, along with most of the trillions of other pointless pictures taken since camera work did really did  become, in the majority of cases, a simple 'point and shoot' exercise. What I do remember was my feeling of pride at my achievement at having made the climb. Everything is relative.

At the hotel in Cordoba, we were assigned to a table with another couple. This presented me with a difficulty I was to face on numerous occasions in the times ahead. What should I tell them? My speech was still a dire mess throughout the Millennium year, as it was to be for long after. I didn't want people to think I was impolite and anyway my inclination is to be sociable. On the other hand, I didn't want anyone to think I was too much of an idiot as soon as I opened my mouth.

What I decided to do was to say something about my difficulties as soon as I could. This has always proved to be the best policy. Over the years, I have been pleasantly surprised at the positive and helpful response of almost everyone. In 2011, when I had to face the same problem once again, it was made far easier for me by the 'speech card' given to me early in the year by Stephanie Godfrey, my speech therapist (see section 24, page 115 and appendix 8, page 157).

She asked me what wording I wanted. I chose '*I have a speech difficulty, but I can understand*'. To me, this means '*I may sound like an idiot but I'm not one*'. Almost always, I get the response as if it had said exactly that, which is heartening to me. I reproduce the image of this card, along with a copy of the one I had made for me by my brother-in-law in Malaysia soon afterwards, in appendix to which I refer.

In fact, I have a number of these laminated cards. This is not so much because wear and tear inevitably take their toll, but because I always keep one in my pocket. Sometimes, I forget to remove them when changing my clothes and have found their appearance is not improved by being put through a washing machine.

My brother-in-law Phil in Australia noticed the success of my speech card and asked me what it said. Before I showed him, I told him the one I used in Australia said, '*I'll slip you fifty dollars when he's not looking.*' The cards are worth a lot more than fifty dollars to me.

In Andalusia we did the touristy things: saw the Alhambra Palace and joked about the name of the Generalife Gardens in Granada, looked for the barber's shop in Seville, visited the mosque in Cordoba and so on. My mobility was no real problem, except when I had to go up, and much more so, down steps. At this stage, I did find even fairly gentle exercise tiring. But it was worth it.

It was also good to enjoy the more casual pleasures of a drink or snack in a pavement café, something we are not permitted to do often enough in the UK because of our wayward climate.

My strongest memory of the week in Spain was supplied by the swimming pool of our Cordoba hotel. After some thought, I decided to go in for a dip. It may have been early days but isn't swimming often used as a form of physical therapy? This was the way my reasoning went. So, I entered the pool.

I was surprised to find I couldn't swim face down. My right side had been weakened (fortunately, it's almost entirely recovered since) and the water made me flip over. This was disconcerting and made me feel vulnerable. Fortunately, I could still swim on my back; though soon found I was travelling in small anti-clockwise circles. I stayed in the pool only for about ten minutes on that first venture.

There were some hairy moments during that week. I found it difficult to come *down* the steps in the front of our Cordoba hotel and it was alarming to be at the top of a steel flight of stairs in a split-level coach station at which we stopped. Objectively, I could now understand why the insurance companies refused to take on anyone within six months of a serious illness. But I had learned much about how to manage my new life in Spain.

At the end of a week we flew back to Cardiff Airport. Our flight home was timed for an hour later than those of most of our fellow holidaymakers, who were returning to various airports in England. We'd enjoyed our time in Spain, and as we bid farewell to everyone, I knew, whatever else it might do, my illness at least wouldn't confine me to the United Kingdom.

## [10] Goodbye to All That Work

Work, or at any rate employment, which is not quite the same thing, has never been at the centre of my Universe. This is as well because I had to give it up, quite literally, overnight.

Don't get me wrong; I knew it was an *important* part of what I did. Anything taking up so much of a life has to be a key part of it, leaving aside all the factors like the social aspects, status and even basic things like food and shelter that are part of the package. It can be interesting to sit down for a moment and work out roughly how much of one's time is taken up by employment. In my own case a crude calculation would have been something like:

| Activity | Hours p.w. | % |
|---|---|---|
| Employment | 40 | 24 |
| Sleep | 49 | 29 |
| Travel etc. to work | 12 | 7 |
| Other Personal Work | 20 | 12 |
| Leisure, Everything Else | 47 | 27 |

*['Personal work' here means attending to life's essentials]*

Individuals will argue that these figures don't apply to them. They will say they need more or less than seven hours sleep a night, that they spend a lot more or less than forty hours in work, that their travel times are vastly greater and so on. Of course, they will be right. The actual working time figure I have given is probably far too modest for me and travelling certainly took up a bigger slice of my day when I worked in Cardiff than when I worked locally.

The essential point is that, unless they are employed part-time or not at all, or are otherwise occupied, few people will spend much less than a quarter of their lives engaged in the various activities surrounding employment.

By the year 2000, I had risen to a moderately senior position in local government. It is currently fashionable to deride any kind of public sector employment, but I had a busy job and worked hard. I knew my efforts were appreciated and I consider that I gave, in the popular phrase, 'value for money'. I think this was true of most of my earlier employment – I've had a wide variety of it. Nor, on the whole, did I mind what I did. There were many aspects of my employment I actually liked throughout my working life, not only when the Millennium year arrived.

There were 'high points' even among the lowest times. I consider my working life has enriched me in all sorts of ways. The various things I have done to earn a living have mostly suited my outlook at the time. I certainly can't put any claim to ever having any kind of grand 'life plan' that meant much. This is simply the way it was.

So, whilst an important part of my days vanished in the Millennium year, fortunately I don't think a hole was punched through the middle of my life – by having to give up work, at least.

I have seen many people, even after a normal, anticipated retirement, struggling to come to terms with their changed situations and am pleased to say this didn't apply to me. On my fifty-second birthday, I didn't see retirement as being just around the corner. I was vaguely looking forward to the years ahead when I'd have the freedom to do what I wanted. I occasionally anticipated with pleasure the liberty that would be mine after retirement in something like 5-10 years after it turned out to be in the event. But I had been giving the prospect no serious thought beyond this.

Edmund was still in his first undergraduate year and Joseph was two years behind him. Suki and I had planned for the expense of their higher education so this wasn't really a major factor in the year 2000 when my unexpected retirement suddenly arrived. Still, this was one more thing that had been keeping retirement off my near horizon.

I knew as early as April 2000 when I was still in hospital I'd almost certainly have to give up my employment, though was in no particular hurry to go through the formalities until I was absolutely sure which way the land was lying. I had personal visits from colleagues and from the occupational doctor and large numbers of letters and cards from those who had worked with me recently and not-so-recently. These did me a power of good, as I describe in Section [7], page 39.

After a few months, a group of my more immediate colleagues got together to have a pub lunch with me once a month. This practice we regularly enjoyed for a number of years, until one-by-one my dining companions moved on to pastures new, either by retiring themselves, moving overseas or both. Take a bow Allan, Geoff, Janet, Jenny, Nyall and Richard.

I don't believe I've undergone much, if anything, of a personality change by having to give up work, nor indeed by any aspect of my illnesses. True, the 'responsibilities of office' had been lifted from my shoulders, but I'd always done my best to carry them lightly. I always made a conscious effort not let them get too much in the way of what I wanted to do.

One of my more savage jokes (I have a weakness for these, sorry) is 'I can't say I've stared death in the face. I was asleep at the time.' This may not be in good taste, but it's true enough.

My income was more than halved when I suddenly retired. This was not something for which I'd planned but was not the disaster you might think it was. I've always lived a modest lifestyle (I dignify this by claiming to be non-materialistic) and had no significant debts at the time of my ill-health retirement. And there were compensations. Along with the drastic pecuniary reduction came a corresponding increase in the hours I could think of as my own property.

To start with I simply wasn't well enough to make the most of this newfound freedom but, after necessarily concentrating on the immediate demands of recovery, I found I could start thinking of my life as my own again. What I've tried to do with it I describe in Section [28], page 135.

There were – still are – all sorts of constraints upon me, but I have learned to cope with these, if not wholly to accept them.

Still, one must never accept too much.

## [11] New York, New York

In the late spring of 2001 Edmund told us he'd applied for a job in the summer following completion of his second university year. This was to be in New York, where he'd be working in the gift shop underneath the Statue of Liberty. We were pleased when he informed us soon afterwards he'd been successful with his application, though could not have been as delighted as he was himself. He was ready to be on his way as soon as end-of-year commitments allowed.

In June, Suki and I made the sudden decision that we'd like to go to visit him. Suki was working at the time, but we calculated we'd be able to squeeze in five days during July. Joseph was finishing his A-levels. Naturally, the prospect of delaying his eighteenth birthday meal for a month to enjoy one in New York during July appealed to him.

Our accommodation was in a hotel in 45th Street. It was high-priced but hardly brilliant, with overworked and unhelpful staff. Still, what else could we expect in the centre of the great city? We only really needed a sleeping base. The five days of our visit were packed with activity. My recovery was still at an early stage and I was tired by our demanding schedule, but glad to be. I was happy to grab a few hours' rest in our room when I could.

We took a cruise on the Hudson River, walked through Central Park and Greenwich Village, and went to the top of the Empire State Building. The World Trade Centre was still standing in that July, but we decided we'd prefer to ascend the older famous tall building. Joseph's eighteenth birthday meal, shared by the four of us, was in a quiet street in 'Little Italy'. It was late at night because of Edmund's work commitments: he was working on the ferry crew transporting goods to Liberty Island as well as in the gift shop. The highlight of our short holiday, though, came on our first full day in the City.

On the day before, our flight into JFK airport had been without incident and, save for a short delay while the baggage conveyor broke down, so was the dreary but brief and efficient process of going through the entry formalities. These were still brief and efficient at that time.

It wouldn't have been that way for the millions being 'processed' through the halls of Ellis Island in the latter part of the nineteenth and first quarter of the twentieth centuries. Their entry to the 'land of the free', ironically close to the Statue of Liberty, was altogether different. We were to learn this emphatically on the island.

Three of us made the short sea-trip to Ellis by the ferry 'Miss Liberty'. The weather was glorious; the sun shone brightly, and the waters of the harbour were calm. I managed the embarkation with no particular difficulty, even though I had to take great care because of my double vision; falling into the water didn't feature in my plans. I had still not grown used to my diplopia (over subsequent years I was to discover you never quite do this) and looking down at New York Harbour from the upper deck gave a distinctly surreal impression.

The ferry docked briefly at Liberty Island, where the majority of our fellow-passengers disembarked. We didn't get off the boat ourselves. The guidebooks told of long queues and the message had been reinforced by Edmund, who was, as he described it, 'selling tat' in the gift shop at the base of the statue at that very moment. Instead, we stayed aboard and went on to Ellis Island. We were glad we'd decided on this minority plan. It was still fairly early in the morning when we reached our destination. To start our visit by being among the first of the day's many visitors gave a false but welcome impression of having the place to ourselves.

Because of the vast oyster banks which are a feature of New York Bay, it used to be called Oyster Island by the Dutch and Gull Island by the Canarsee Indians before them. The final name was given for Samuel Ellis, an eighteenth-century landowner. It was leased by the City of New York, which in turn sold it to the federal government, even though there was some dispute about its title. This built the reception centre to replace the small Castle Garden (Kestelgartel) in 1892.

Today the island, restored to its early 20th century condition, is a free and rather special museum telling the story of the 'huddled masses' who had come to the land where they would supposedly be at liberty to carve out a future for their families. The majority of them were to find that earlier settlers had already carved out most of the best bits for themselves.

The hopeful new Americans had already endured long sea-voyages with sparse diets like constant potatoes and salted herrings before stepping ashore for their medical and financial examination, then a quick-fire questioning session from an inspector. Many of the newcomers, in fact, spent only a matter of hours or at most a day or two on the island before going on to America proper.

The feared thing for an immigrant was to have 'SI' (for 'Special Investigation') recorded against his or her name. This was usually for a suspected medical problem like trachoma or tuberculosis. An initial would also be chalked on the unfortunate person's sleeve signifying there was to be a more detailed examination or inquiry. The worst outcome was to be shipped back to the port of origin. This happened in two or three per cent of cases. This may have been a small proportion, but it represented a large number of people.

The museum concentrates on these detainees (there were well over a quarter of a million of them) and is an eerie reminder of today's refugees and the difficult issues faced by receiving Governments. It tells its story by a successful mix of modern technology and artefacts of the time and is housed in a building of quietly stunning architecture.

The harassed officials baptised so many American citizens here. Irving Berlin came as Israel Beilin and Samuel Goldwyn was originally Ben Shahn. There is a story that an old Russian Jew had failed to remember the 'American-sounding' name he had intended to give and could only mutter in Yiddish that he'd forgotten - *Schon vergessen*. He was registered as John Ferguson.

Our visit ended with lunch, bought earlier in a Manhattan deli, and eaten overlooking New York harbour. We were sitting on the grass and free to leave by the next boat, or the one after. The immigrants who were here in the last century wouldn't have had this choice.

It was still a beautiful day and we'd all found our visit to be rewarding. I would recommend that you go, too, if you ever find yourself in this lively city. I don't think I'd like to go to Ellis Island again, though, much as I enjoyed this visit. And I understand why most of those who entered America through Ellis Island wouldn't have wanted to go there again, either.

*

About two months later, on 11<sup>th</sup> September, to be exact, I was sitting at home. Joseph was with me, spending a pleasant few week of idleness, while waiting for his own turn to begin university toward the end of the month. Suki was with

Debbie, our next-door neighbour.

We were surprised when Suki rang to tell us to put on the television. We did and were stunned with the news that a jet aeroplane had crashed into the World Trade Centre. Minutes later, there were live pictures of the second jet crashing into the building. At first sight I thought it was a particularly tasteless advertising stunt. As the drama painfully continued, I knew it couldn't be.

My life was not the only one to be changed early in the new Millennium. It gave me a different perspective on my own problems. With the ugly turn the world took in 2001, the life of everyone on our planet has altered for the worse in some way. Our world is still not running straight and true. This is in large part due to the events of 11<sup>th</sup> September, 2001, though more recent events have given us a further kick in the teeth. Nobody will need me to describe them but see the final section on page 137.

Our first thoughts were for Edmund, naturally. The World Trade Centre and the Statue of Liberty were close together. We knew our son's schedule should have taken him to see a friend in Iowa by around 11th September. We e-mailed him but didn't get a reply straight away; in the event he was still in transit from New York. This we were unsure of at the time. What if he'd changed his plans? We were mightily relieved to get an e-mail from him the next day.

He was due to fly home a few days later, but all flights out of the USA were grounded. Later, he told us internal as well as external transport was thrown into confusion. This was why he didn't at first receive our email; he had indeed needed to change his travel plans. His visit to Iowa was briefer than planned and it wasn't easy for him to make his way back to New York. Eventually, he was able to do so and, after spending a night on a friend's floor, managed to board one of the first transatlantic flights.

Although we originally had no plans to greet him at the airport, Joseph and I went to meet him at Gatwick. Wouldn't you have done the same?

## [12] Lessons on The Rhine

Although we'd ventured to New York in the previous year, I was still far from recovered by 2002. Nevertheless, we decided to go on an overseas holiday again. We chose carefully, settling on a Rhine river cruise. Our thought was that, in this way, we'd be able to see a fair bit of the German countryside but at the same time would have a permanent cabin for the week and so dispense with the slog of constantly packing and unpacking. This would have been too much like hard work for me at that stage.

The early indications were not promising. In 2002, I still needed an hour's bed rest in the afternoon. On our first full day on the river, my 'down time' coincided with a routine fire drill. We were supposed to assemble at a specified point on deck when the alarm bell rang. I didn't stir. Although I knew what I was hearing might just have been the bell sounding for a real fire and not a drill, I was simply too weary to get out of bed when the alarm sounded.

The crew were conscientious. When I failed to appear one of them knocked and opened my door. When she saw me supine, she told me to stay where I was. At the time I was grateful for this but later wasn't so pleased with myself. More than anything, this was because I was dissatisfied with what it told me about my rate of recovery.

An hour or two afterwards, I went up to the top deck of the boat, the back part of which had been set aside for entertainment and diversions. There was a woman on an exercise bike, some years older than me, I'd suppose (though probably not older than I am now!) For a long time, she kept up a steady pedalling.

Anyone could see the illness she'd suffered had left physical marks upon her. Her right leg had clearly been weakened and her right eye was drooping markedly. It looked very much as if she were recovering from a stroke. She saw me looking and smiled, then resumed pedalling all the harder. My own illness had left me with no obvious health problems. Unless they spoke to me or observed me descending stairs, no one would even have guessed I'd been ill. I felt ashamed of myself in comparison with this lady and resolved to get my act together.

That evening, we shared our dinner table with an elderly couple from London. His name was George; I can't remember hers. I discovered that, years before, he'd been the chief trainer for an amateur boxing club in Shoreditch, in the East End of London. He'd devoted many hours to it and clearly regretted having to recount his experience in the past tense.

I'd had an interest in boxing myself from the late nineteen-fifties until the mid-eighties when, at least at the top level and thanks to the new breed of promoters, the sport transformed itself into a shoddy branch of show business. I don't know what made me think of it, but suddenly I recalled the name of a talented lightweight I knew came from Hoxton, close to Shoreditch. He used to be a professional boxer in the nineteen-sixties and so might have been an amateur during George's era.

'Do you remember Vic Andreetti?' I asked.

The effect on George was immediate. He spluttered, almost choking on his dinner. His wife, a concerned, pleasant lady was clearly worried for a moment. But George quickly recovered and couldn't have been more delighted with my question. It turned out he'd been Vic Andreetti's senior trainer and mentor as an amateur. George also regarded himself as the boxer's chief confidante and had closely followed his professional boxing career. The rest of the evening, indeed our dinners for the remainder of the week, went very well.

*

On the next morning, or it may have been the day after, we moored near the *Stollwerck* chocolate factory and museum at Cologne. I enjoyed our morning visit to the works, where we bought a few bars to take home with us. Still, Suki and Joseph could probably sense my eagerness to get on with the main event of the day, later on in the morning. For it was then we were due to go to the Beer Festival.

Our courier on the *Regina Rheni*, the 'Queen of the Rhine', had quite casually mentioned the fact that there was a beer festival in the cathedral city while we were there. It was almost like an afterthought on his part.  If this was in deference to the mature years of most of the passengers (we were well below the average age of those on this cruise; I enjoyed the illusions this provided!) he need not have bothered. Many of the passengers went to the festival in the morning. A number of them stayed all day.

I hadn't been to a beer festival for many years. The only previous occasion was in my youth, somewhere in England. If this sounds a little vague to you, this is because my memories of the day are rather blurry. In fact, they were rather blurry by the next day or even later on the same day.

My approach at Cologne was to be rather different to the sink 'em down one I'd employed more than thirty years before. Because of the company I was in, and because I was supposedly, though questionably, more mature in outlook, as well as the fact that I was still in the early stages of recovery, I knew I'd have to slow down a bit this time.

I decided to look upon my visit as a variation of a wine-tasting. This was the theory, at any rate. I knew it wouldn't be exactly like a wine tasting, where the tendency is too often for people to pretend they know more than they really do, and to treat what should be an enjoyable drink with far too much reverence. But you will get my drift.

When we came to the beer festival site, we found that the exhibits were housed in what reminded me more than anything else of fairground stalls. There were large, and sometimes small, circular wooden constructions. The look of the site didn't auger well for my resolve to treat the exercise as a freewheeling, though still decorous, variant of wine tasting.

Following our pre-agreed plan, we first made a more or less complete circuit of the grounds. The exhibits consisted of a hundred or so beer-stalls, a half dozen or more eating places, some seating, and two stages for the entertainment, to be provided by oom-pa-pa style bands. But all the time I was anxious to make my first purchase. The yeast was entering my soul.

My knowledge of the German language is rudimentary to say the least (there's no false modesty here). I can stutter out things like '*Drei schwarzbier bitte*' and '*Zwei bier und eine kaffee bitte*' but beyond that I am severely taxed. It was a good job there weren't four of us. I was nevertheless appointed the unofficial interpreter; my wife and son knew even less German than I did. Still, I was to find that '*bitteschön*' and '*dankeschön*' to the accompaniment of an extended, if shaky, index finger will get you a long way.

It was a shame we'd booked to return to the *Regina Rheni* for lunch, because the sausages we tried were simply delicious. I hardly know my knackwurst from my frankfurters (isn't one of them a smoked sausage?) but this hardly mattered. We just followed our noses, and the stall keepers followed my pointed index finger.

It doesn't take much of a genius to work out that I visited a number of beer stalls. When we returned in the afternoon, I hadn't managed to visit all one hundred stalls, but dark beer, wheat beer, cloudy beer and even a few lager-like beers all went down the same way. I had never been to a wine tasting like this. My favourite tipple turned out to be something not far different from the *Kristall Weizen* available in our local supermarkets. Oh well.

By late afternoon, my forefinger was getting wobblier and my precarious hold on German had become even shakier. The faces of the jolly stall holders became even jollier. We made an erratic return to the boat without so much as stepping inside Cologne's great cathedral, although it was only yards from the festival. Never mind. I had made devotions enough.

*

Returning to *Regina Rheni*, I slept. This was to be the last of my daily naps. I awoke an hour or so before the time of our evening meal quite refreshed and not much the worse for wear. The dinner was very tasty, as indeed dinners were for the whole week. I asked George how he had spent his own day.

'Why, we went to the beer festival, of course', he said, clearly surprised by my question. 'It was extraordinarily good.' And for a moment he was lost in his thoughts.

'He's incorrigible, isn't he?' said his wife.

Then she astounded us by saying that George was no less than ninety-two years old, while she was eighty-nine. I worked out that, when I went to that English beer festival what seemed like all those years before, George would have been older than I was in 2002.

## [13] On the Road

One immediate result of my first haemorrhage was that I could no longer drive.

In most cases, there is a legal requirement to tell the DVLA when you have suffered a stroke. The Department published a leaflet which, in the variety of semi-legalese reserved for Government publications, at that time said you should advise them if '*One month after the stroke you are still suffering from weakness of the arms or legs, visual disturbance, or problems with co-ordination, memory or understanding*'.

My recovery was already proceeding at an encouraging pace by the summer of the year 2000 when I had my first tentative look at this. I could probably have made a case for driving on most of these points (not that I was in a great hurry to do that) but there was no doubt that my 'visual disturbances' were severe at that stage. They still are.

I filled in the alarming DVLA questionnaire, providing them with consultant and physiotherapist details and sent with it a medical letter as soon as October 2000, even though I had no intention of driving at what I considered to be still an early stage. My thought was simply to prepare the groundwork for later.

Many people would have found the loss of freedom given by driving to be a damaging thing. I can't honestly say I did. It was certainly an inconvenience. This is hardly the same.

When I worked for an employer in Cardiff, it was more or less essential for me to drive to carry out certain of my duties. It wasn't strictly necessary for making the forty-mile round trip for commuting. Then, rail services weren't as overcrowded as they are now, and I always preferred to travel by train. I found it infinitely more relaxing to start the day by having a chat with friends and colleagues than to suffer the tedium of rush hour road travel to Central Cardiff. In 1996, my employment moved to my hometown. Driving, whilst still useful in my job, then became inessential.

Of course, driving was also important in my personal life. Apart from holiday and other purely leisure purposes, I was used to being able to make many journeys by road in connection with my interest in writing. To give just one example, it was easy to be able to jump in the car and go off to speak to someone (to 'interview them', I suppose I should say, though I could never think of it in those terms) whose business was the focus of a commercial feature. These were one of the dimensions of my writing interest at that time. After my first illness, these interviews became less easy to carry out at exactly the time that commercial features became more important to me.

All the same, there were some plus points to the changes forced upon me. My friend Ewart was always willing and indeed keen to drive me to places. I think he liked the process as well as the result. Our wives most often were with us and we four would make a morning of it, with lunch afterwards.

Suki would take notes for me (I'd lost the ability to write swiftly in longhand) and Ewart would take some useful photographs. He was skilful with his camera and to use it with a definite purpose was a thing that appealed to him. I appreciated it greatly to have my own photographer with me instead of a camera!

A single instance of the old and new arrangements in action will best serve to illustrate the changes. One afternoon in the late nineties I took a half-day's leave from work to make the hundred-mile round trip to the Brecon area with the intention of talking to the owner of the new Welsh whisky distillery. While I was at it, I took a few photographs. It was an interesting experience, as most of them were, and the resulting feature appeared in an airline magazine. Welsh whisky was a novel idea at the time.

Unfortunately, despite opening a visitor's centre and looking set for a bright future, the business didn't prosper. The process of distilling takes time. It has to be a long-term project and must be financed during the initial period when no compensating revenue from sales of the product can be expected. The company struggled through this period and eventually went into liquidation.

However, soon afterwards some enterprising South Walians had the idea (over a chat in a pub, I was told!) of trying again, this time on a on a more ambitious scale. The clear focus was to be on whisky actually distilled in Wales. There was no serious initial thought of becoming a tourist attraction.

The Welsh Whisky Company duly opened early in this Millennium in Penderyn, a village at the southern edge of the Brecon Beacons National Park. With careful planning, the company survived the difficult early period. The single malt Penderyn Whisky went on sale for the first time in 2004; on St David's day as you might expect. It was the first time that whisky had been distilled in Wales since 1906. The venture at the end of the previous Millennium hadn't got to the stage of making saleable whisky. On this occasion, it was to be different. The vital time for maturation had been factored in.

When I heard of the new company's early efforts, I arranged to go to Penderyn in March, 2005. The Managing Director, Stephen Davies, spoke at length to me, answered my many questions and showed us all around the distillery. What he thought when four of us turned up and when he found my speech wasn't quite normal were things I didn't care to ask. I should, however, say that he treated me with courtesy and was highly informative and forthcoming. He also gave the four of us a taste of whisky!

Ewart took some excellent photographs for me and, with the aid of Suki's comprehensive notes; it was plain sailing to put together a feature. This appeared in a magazine only a few months after our visit to Penderyn. It amused me when the editor of the magazine added this 'blurb' underneath the title (I'd called the piece 'The Spirit of Wales'): '*It's a hard job but someone has to do it. (Tom East) downs the challenge to discover the wonders of Welsh whisky.*' I tried to keep quiet about the fact that I'd always preferred brandy.

In 2005, when I visited, The Welsh Whisky Company was just getting off the ground. At that stage there was no visitor centre, nor yet any definite plans to build one. The company's attention was fixed firmly on its priority of actually distilling whisky. However, even at that stage, there was forming an outline idea for a centre. This was duly opened in 2008, in the presence of Prince Charles.

Since those early days, the company has gone from strength to strength. Penderyn Whisky now has an international reputation. Suki and I took a bottle as a gift for our brother-in-law Phil when we visited him and his wife Wanda (Suki's sister) in Western Australia in 2017, only to find it was on sale in the local supermarket

I see that around the time I wrote *The Spirit of Wales* I also placed several other commercial features. Three of these involved excursions for 'the gang of four'. In two, Ewart's photographic skills rather than my eccentric interviewing technique or his own driving were the key factors. In the fourth, it was useful to be able to make the long journey to the one of the boatyards on a local canal to speak to the owner. So, my problems with driving weren't wholly bad news, in this respect at least.

For a long time after March, 2000, my car spent most of its time in the garage. I didn't touch the steering wheel for the next two years. My neighbour, Peter, took the car and ourselves out for a spin now and again, so as to prevent the battery from going flat. These included, one day, making the 190-mile round trip to Fishguard.

A number of friends were happy to give me lifts to other places. It is easy to reach the centre of my town, from where good public transport links are available. But, by 2002, I was keen to resume driving, at least locally. By that time, I had DVLA approval to take the wheel. Peter was brave enough to take me to the quiet roads of our local industrial estate to see how I'd get on with driving the car.

I managed well enough and resumed driving. I say 'managed', but I was never entirely happy on the road after the year 2000. My self-driven car journeys never reached beyond the local area. My range was limited to the weekly supermarket shopping and a few short leisure trips.

Before long, I found that the easiest way to cope with my double vision was simply to close my left eye when making a manoeuvre like taking a corner or going on a roundabout, when it became necessary for me to move my head more than a little. Any car driver will tell you it's essential to move your head when driving!

One occasion remains vivid in my mind. I was driving my sons to a local swimming pool. Edmund, who was at that time between two overseas employments in Japan and China, was unfamiliar with my unusual cornering technique. He was sitting to my left in the front passenger seat.

'Are you all right, Dad?' he asked in alarm, as I closed my left eye in my usual way of taking a left-hand corner. Of course, it looked to him from my left-hand side as if I were shutting *both* eyes to perform the manoeuvre. We all laughed uproariously when we discussed the matter, but the incident stuck in my mind.

Many people assume I stopped driving when I had my second haemorrhage. This wasn't so. I'd thought about what I should do for most of the decade. It was a relief to sell the car in January 2010. By then I'd qualified for free bus travel and frequently use the good service we have to travel to town. But I still like to walk the mile-and-a-third when the weather allows it, as well as taking longer walks. Now I have a pedometer instead of a car!

I haven't given a moment's serious thought to driving since the day I sold my car.

## [14] Walking and Talking

My early progress with the more physical problems was highly satisfying. Before the first year had passed I could walk significant distances and, although it remained difficult to use my right hand with any accuracy and my double vision remained a problem, I could also claim to have regained nearly all of my bodily attributes.

Not so my speech. This was a real struggle. As the year 2000 passed into the year 2001 I accepted there was going to be no help from formal speech therapy. I was on my own. Still, I reasoned that it would have been primarily down to my own efforts in any event. My thinking was that much practice was going to be necessary. This is the way it proved to be.

Aphasia (sometimes called dysphasia), where the communication centres of the brain are damaged, is a common legacy of strokes and haemorrhages. It can affect things like understanding, vocabulary, and other aspects of the ability to handle language. Fortunately for me, in my own case purely speech was affected.

Something like this is only to be expected, if you think of it for a moment. Speaking, which most of us are able to take for granted, is in reality one of the more complex actions we do. It demands coordinated effort from the intellectual, speech and language centres in the brain and the motor centres (which do things like moving the tongue and lips in a precise and delicate way and help with control of the breath).

A brain haemorrhage destroys some of the neural pathways, the nerve connections between the various parts of the brain and to other parts of our bodies. It can also adversely affect the channels within the central nervous system. To have any chance of repairing these functions, the brain therefore has to forge alternate paths, a large number of which are required for speaking. The new ones cannot be as effective as the ones we've formed throughout our lives, from infancy onwards.

In effect, at least to some degree, it is necessary to learn to talk over again as we did in our early years. And our brains aren't as adaptable as they were when we were in our early years.

I decided the only way forward was going to be to try to, quite literally, talk through the difficulty as best I was able. This wasn't easy. One of the things I had been able to do reasonably well in my previous life was speak. Talking in public held no undue fears for me.

In my employment over a period ten or so years, along with a series of colleagues, I ran a course on speaking in public. We called it *Training the Trainers*. Its ostensible purpose was to prepare tutors for our internal training programme. In reality, its aim was bolder. It was aimed at decreasing the 'fear factor' that can be a concomitant of any kind of public- or semi-public speaking.

In the dozen years before my haemorrhage, my interest in creative writing had been reawakened. It was something I enjoyed and which gave me much satisfaction. To me, the written word was always *the* thing but there is no doubt that support from the author's spoken word is also not far off indispensable.

It is an irony that, on the *Training the Trainer* courses, I'd always recommend that the speaker's notes should be in bullet or key point form. My argument was that this retained the spontaneity of the spoken word. This would be lost if a script were written out for reading in full.

In the only public speaking I did after the year 2000, I needed to read out things (usually poetry) for which I had the complete text before me. It must be that I needed the neural pathways and couldn't waste them too much on mere thinking! At least, especially in the early years of recovery, I found it next-to-impossible to read or talk and think at the same time.

Despite all the difficulties, I remained keen to be able to regain some ability to read in public again. This as well, of course, as recovering the ability to do simple things like speaking reasonably coherently to friends and family. One result of my difficulties was that, in trying to make myself understood, I tended to say things with slightly more force than I'd want. I am so grateful to people (nearly everyone, fortunately) who was and is prepared to tolerate my excesses.

I also find it preferable to do simple things like going into a shop and to say what is required without the assistant looking at me as if I'd walked in and uttered that well-known Martian phrase 'take me to your leader'. When going up to a bar, I nowadays make a point of producing my 'speech card' in case I am met with the response 'you've had enough already'!

Some would say I tried to read publicly too soon, but there would never have been a right time. I am a firm believer in the maxim that you have to play the game with the cards you've actually been dealt, not those you wish you held or thought you once did and, if you're very lucky, might hold of again.

The first time I recall reading anything in front of an audience was actually the singing of a song in Port Talbot. I remember the evening well. *The Battle Hymn of the None of the Above Party*, the lyric of mine I chose, went to the theme tune of the old TV series *The Adventures of Robin Hood,* and featured the shuffled names of two politicians. For the purposes of the song, the two main party leaders of the time became 'William Blair' and 'Tony Hague'.

It was actually slightly easier to sing than read; presumably something about the rhythm helps. And, particularly at that stage, I did need a lot of assistance. In fact, my main help on that occasion came not from the rhythms of the song but in the form of my friend Chris, who became my partner in a duet. He also gave me a lift to Port Talbot and, although no-one could describe him as shy, I swear he blanched when his companion, who at that time could hardly string a sentence together, put the proposal for this joint enterprise to him on the way in the car. I call what we presented a 'duet', although in reality the main voice heard on that evening was the one belonging to Chris. Nevertheless, I'd seen my part of it through.

A few months later I pulled exactly the same trick with another friend, Phil. The song was the same, but this time we were in Swansea with a bigger audience. Again, I couldn't claim that mine was the main voice to be heard on that evening. I suppose it's too late to apologise to them after all these years, so I'll just say 'Thanks, Chris and Phil. I did at least buy you a pint.' *Didn't I?*

After those early stumbles I eventually went on to read imperfectly, if slightly less imperfectly as time went on, in a large number of venues in South Wales. It was normally my own writing and poetry rather than songs. There was, however, one Red Poets' evening in the Dylan Thomas centre Chris would probably rather forget. I persuaded him to sing with me my 'updated' version of the socialist anthem, *The Red Flag*. I called it *Y Blodyn Pinc*, which means 'The Pink Flower'. You get the picture.

I shouldn't pretend all was plain sailing. On another evening in the Dylan Thomas Centre in Swansea I read, as did Aeronwy Thomas, the daughter of Dylan Thomas, who was there on that occasion. On the way out I complimented her on two of her poems, carefully not mentioning the third. This really didn't say anything except 'I am Dylan's daughter'.

She said she liked the poems I'd read. Then she turned to my friend, who'd also read. 'I liked your *Seven Lies of Man*,' she said. This was one of the poems of my own and I'd read it myself. Chris looks nothing like me. He's tall, weighty, and bearded. I am none of these things!

Another time in Merthyr Tydfil I read a silly piece of verse called *Superman Returns*. This was written with audience participation in mind; I was pleased when people shouted the refrain at the right points and held their arms aloft on cue. The poem was meant to be ironic, although I'm not sure if it achieved this lofty aim. Afterwards another poet, Peter, quietly asked someone if I was French, and who 'Soup Man' was. This seemed to be missing the point. Well, I suppose I was wearing a Breton shirt on that evening!

# Episode Two
## *Not Again!*

## [15] Out of Focus

People who know me always assume my 'episode one' was caused by stress of some kind. I've never suggested this myself. In fact, I don't think it was so. I'm absolutely sure this wasn't the case with episode two.

Not much more than a week before this 'second episode', on 13th November, 2010 to be exact, Suki and I had gone to Cardiff to do some shopping. We had a meal in an Italian restaurant, where we happened to see my friend Chris and his wife Pam. Cardiff was lively because it was the day of one of Wales' autumn rugby internationals. It was a match against South Africa and resulted in a narrow loss for Wales.

I remember the details well because, later in the afternoon, I walked out by myself to Canton, where two friends were having a joint launch of their newly published books. One of these was a collection of poetry and the other of prose. My walking return journey to Cardiff Central railway station took me past the Millennium Stadium late in the match. Although I didn't find out the exact score until I reached home, the loud collective sigh that went up from the stadium as I walked by and the match finished told me all I needed to know about the result.

A little more than a week after this I went to our local town centre with Suki. This was intended to be no more than a minor run to pick up a few things and we decided to travel on the bus rather than walk. When I arrived in the bus station, I felt slightly – no more than slightly – unwell and thought it best to take the same bus back. When I reached home, I took it easy for the rest of the morning and the early part of the afternoon.

Later, I decided to have a look at the prose book – it was a collection of short stories – I'd bought in Cardiff ten days before. I'd read two of the stories and was about to start a third when my eyesight quite suddenly blurred. The sensation was exactly like looking at a sharp image through an optical lens as, say, those on a pair binoculars or camera would have been, and then having it pulled unexpectedly and quickly out of focus.

This peculiar phenomenon lasted for only about four or five seconds before my vision returned to normal. Then, all at once I felt nauseous. I told Suki about this and she rushed to get the 'sickie bowl', a redundant plastic cake-mixing bowl we'd used for our sons when they were toddlers. Now it was my turn to use it and I did, though not copiously. I remained seated for a minute or two to recover then tried to rise from my seat on the couch, only to fall forward to my knees.

I remained in this kneeling position for some seconds and then, despite Suki's protestations, decided I was well enough to go upstairs to use the toilet. Unable to walk normally, I pulled myself step-by-step upstairs and somehow managed to do what I needed to do. This included throwing up for a second time, more heartily this time. After a few minutes' rest, my locomotion downstairs was even more laboured and awkward, but I managed to back myself down the staircase.

Suki was alarmed but I assured her I was starting to feel better and that the problem must have been caused by a sudden attack of food poisoning. I was indeed starting to feel a bit better – the nausea had passed – but in my heart of hearts I knew things were far from right. I hoisted myself back on to the couch and started to watch the television.

There was a recording of a quiz programme playing – one of the more demanding ones like 'Mastermind' or 'University Challenge' and, as I normally do, I started to give the answers aloud when I knew them. Suki told me afterwards that she was monitoring me carefully at this point and noted I was giving a normal quota of correct answers.

Nevertheless, as the programme went on, I noticed that my speech was deteriorating, even though I was trying to articulate with care. I still tried to convince myself that this must have been due to the food poisoning or whatever it was but deep down, knew this was unlikely to be true. It came to the point where Suki would accept my protestations no longer and ordered me upstairs, then shepherded me into bed. Still I was trying to argue that I was in the throes of an attack of food poisoning.

Even though I didn't really believe this myself, I made her ring our general practitioner's surgery instead of an ambulance.

One of the doctors came fairly quickly. I was able to deal with his questions and answer lucidly but I was aware my power of speech was becoming increasingly difficult to command. The deciding factor for Dr Overton was the fact that I couldn't stand up unaided. He was kind enough not to use the word 'stroke'. He said, 'we'd better get you into hospital, to see what the problem is.' But the three of us already knew what the problem was, even if none of us voiced it.

It was another thirty minutes before the ambulance arrived. By this time, I had struggled downstairs again. I couldn't have looked too bad because one of the ambulance crew asked me if I could walk. He soon found out I couldn't. His colleagues brought in a stretcher.

'He's none too clever on his legs,' were the exact words of his explanation to the others. This was something of an understatement.

It was 23rd November, 2010, the date of my sixty-third birthday.

## [16] Emergency Admission

Unconsciousness had left me with no memories of my previous journey to the A&E unit in the Millennium year. My only other personal experience of the place had been a dozen years before that when I experienced a spectacularly bloody accident to my fingernail. Then I was able to drive myself to the hospital, swaddled finger sticking out crazily. I was even able to drive next day to Warwick in a similar fashion for a family weekend, although this time with a better tied bandage.

In 2010, I was fully conscious but, even if I'd still had a car, there'd have been no prospect of me driving myself. This journey was in an ambulance. Contrary to the many reports we've heard recently of chaotic waiting in hospital emergency waiting units, I didn't have to wait for hours in a corridor or on the ambulance. We were parked outside for only a short time before I was wheeled in on a trolley. My 'processing' was dealt with efficiently. Soon I found myself in a large room with many beds and patients. There was also a good number of medical staff who seemed to be going about their business quickly and efficiently.

The routine medical tests like blood pressure checks, taking samples, temperature and so forth were dealt with without fuss. Nor did I have to wait long to see a doctor. In fact, I saw two. I was able to answer all their questions without too much difficulty, even though I could tell my power of speech was deteriorating further. Indeed, I found I could get out of the hospital bed to perform some simple movements as instructed and to perform similar tasks, even though I couldn't stand without the support of the bed.

Eventually, as I knew would happen, the doctors told me they suspected a bleed and that I was going to be sent for a brain scan. A porter wheeled me off for this. Scans are performed in a large, intimidating cylinder. With minimal assistance, I was able to transfer myself from trolley to scanner bed. This slowly slides in and out of the machine, to the accompaniment of noises that might have come straight from the soundtrack of a second-rate science-fiction film.

Before the scanner starts, the patient is provided with some eye-protection. To me personally, this is the part of the process that fills me with the greatest alarm. As well as making sure the eye-protection is in place, my reaction is to screw my eyes as tightly shut as I can. Even then, I'm intensely aware of a variety of flashes intruding on my senses, making me feel helpless and vulnerable. Objectively, I'd have to say that the whole process is dealt with speedily, but objectivity is hard to achieve in these circumstances.

Not many minutes later I was back in the A&E unit, awaiting the result of the scan. I didn't have to wait long. A young doctor, whose name I've unfortunately forgotten, came to tell me I had indeed experienced a cerebral haemorrhage.

This was in the cerebellum, she told me. This is the 'small brain' underneath the main hemispheres. I'd touched on the study of brain anatomy in my degree course years before – one thing I recalled doing was dissecting a sheep's brain – and was aware that the cerebellum was the centre of certain functions, such as balance and 'over-learned activities' like riding a bicycle and playing music.

I'd never learned to play a musical instrument but could appreciate the balance problem, currently having first-hand experience of it. Trying to stand up was an alarming experience.

In 2000, the bleeding had been in quite another area of my brain, the left-hand frontal cortex. This is the centre of a number of higher brain functions, including speech. It had taken me ten-and-a-half years and a great deal of effort to regain a workable standard of speech.

So, although it could hardly be good news to be told I'd suffered another haemorrhage, I reasoned that things could have been worse. I knew the odds against surviving were at least 4/1 (a statistician might explain they were even longer).

This was the way I at first reasoned things out from my hospital bed. Considering everything, I wasn't feeling too bad. I hadn't lost consciousness or lucidity for even a second. I had cautious confidence that I'd be able to recover my balance over time. The new bleed was well away from the main speech area, so some of my current problems might be temporary. This was the bit of information I hung onto grimly. I remembered my previous experience only too well.

It was not to be so simple in practice.

The doctor, a charming Scots young woman who hailed from Inverness, told me she was arranging for my admission to the hospital. Before much longer, I was wheeled off to the ward. This was in semi-darkness; by then the hour was late. All of the other patients in the ward were sleeping or at least lying quietly in their beds. Sleep was not for me; I simply wasn't ready for it. Besides, Suki was still with me and I wanted to try to talk to her, even though my speech problem was getting worse by the minute.

My diminished powers of conversation weren't taxed for long. Not twenty minutes later, the Scots doctor returned to tell me that she'd made enquiries of the specialist neurosurgical ward in the University Hospital of Wales in Cardiff (called by everyone locally 'The Heath'). They had a vacant bed. How did I feel about taking it? She told me my condition was 'good' – I knew what she meant. 'They're the experts,' she added.

I knew my answer could be only 'yes', even though I was unhappy about the word 'neurosurgical'. A surgeon's knife in my brain was not something I was keen to experience. A short time later, I was being wheeled from the ward to another ambulance. Suki came with me. The interior of the ambulance felt chillingly cold and the crew gave me an extra blanket. The temperature on that 23rd November was indeed around freezing point but I felt it all the more because by this time I was, frankly, becoming afraid.

The journey by road between the two hospitals is a straightforward one. It should not have taken much more than half-an-hour. We experienced no traffic hold-ups – it was after all becoming late on a mid-week night – but to me it seemed interminable.

I was anxious to reach our destination even though it was already filling me with nightmare visions. When the ambulance doors opened, I could see the many tall buildings of the hospital, Wales' largest, looming down all about me. It was like finding myself transported to an alien world. This wasn't where I wanted to be. But what choice did I have?

## [17] My Darkest Night

That November night was extraordinarily cold, heralding the early onset of the winter of 2010/11. The first snows were to arrive only a few days later. The weather suited my grim mood as I looked from the back of the ambulance to the grounds of the Heath Hospital.

Without fuss, I was wheeled from the ambulance to the High Dependency Unit of the Neurosurgical Ward. Here, at around midnight, I was installed in a bed next to the window, which was partly open. Despite the draught of cold air thus admitted, this was perfect for me; I wouldn't have liked to be anywhere nearer the centre of the incredibly hot room. A junior doctor, a friendly young man, saw and assessed me soon after my admission, then spoke to the nursing staff to give them instructions. One of the health care assistants took Suki into a side room to have a cup of tea and a nap.

My long night had begun.

The man in the bed opposite had a choking cough. This erupted every ten minutes or so; I could get no sleep. Not that I felt like any. After an hour or so, a nurse drew the curtains around him. Before this, his face had to me looked the picture of abject misery. It was as if he knew he was not long for this world. Nor was he; after a particularly furious bout of coughing, an odd spluttering gurgle came from behind the curtains. Then there was silence.

A few minutes later there was a flurry of medical activity around the bed. Before long, the to-ing and fro-ing became less frenzied and the bed was quietly wheeled out. Another man, in a bed further into the interior of the ward, also died that night. Yet another of my original fellow-patients made his quiet exit a few days later, although by this time I'd been promoted to another unit. On my first night this second patient, for some reason, insisted on rising from his bed all the time. The staff had the Devil's own job in persuading him to take some rest.

Getting out of bed was something I'd have dearly loved to do myself. Instead, I had no escape from the regime of medical checks made by the staff nurse, a Filipina. I saw her only on that one night, so presume she was from a nursing agency. Whether she was or not, she carried out her duties conscientiously, resting her hand reassuringly on my side as she checked my pulse.

Besides the pulse-checking, she made two other checks every fifteen minutes. One was verbal; she'd ask the same two questions each time: *'what year is this?'* and *'who is your prime minister?'* My answers were consistent: *'1927'* and *'same as yours, unfortunately.'* I'm still not sure whether she realised I was trying to inject some sort of levity into the situation. She quite probably couldn't even understand what I was saying. Perhaps she thought I'd flipped. Still, I stuck to my desperate guns throughout the night; I found it impossible to give a straight answer. I was trying to reassure myself I suppose.

The other check was more alarming. After our bizarre question-and-answer session, she'd shine a penlight torch into each of my eyes in turn. Presumably, this was to see if my pupils would contract. I couldn't help but think of it as a check to see if there was anyone at home. This made it frightening when, at about 3am, she called the junior doctor in, as if for a second opinion.

With excruciating slowness, the dark skies turned grey and a few feeble notes of birdsong sounded from the hospital grounds. The other patients began to stir. The nurse and her colleague health care assistant smiled at me. Both advised me to drink plenty of water: *'You want to get out of that, bed, don't you?'* I certainly did. I drank three whole jugs full in short order. My bladder was full to bursting point as I was helped to the toilet.

It would be good to record that the sunbeams broke into the ward to herald the new dawn as I was aided in my trek to the toilet. They didn't. The morning light was sombre. Still, my darkest night was over.

*

Throughout the day I did some catching up on the sleep I'd missed the night before. I even ate a little food; more importantly I obsessively drank more water, necessitating frequent assisted journeys to the loo. Other than a wheelchair journey to the floor below to have another brain scan, the day and following night were uneventful. The investigation only confirmed the diagnosis I had been given in my local hospital of another brain haemorrhage. As they'd thought it was in the cerebellum, underneath the two large hemispherical cortices.

On the Thursday morning I saw the consultant and his team. He patiently explained to me what had happened. I was less than patient when I asked why, if this bleeding had occurred in my cerebellum, my speech had been so severely affected? I could understand if it meant I wouldn't be able to play the piano (I'd never been able to do this anyway) but I understood the speech centres weren't located in the cerebellum. With even more patience he explained (paraphrasing), that it wasn't quite as simple as that, and the brain functions aren't organised into neat boxes with little labels attached to them.

*

Later that day I was moved to a side room. This was for ward convenience, not for any medical reason. In fact, my condition was improving. I was able to send my sons, who lived some miles away in different towns, a text message to tell them what had happened, where I was, and to say that their mother would ring them later with more details. It wasn't easy to manipulate the small mobile phone keyboard, but I was putting into action the plan I had discussed with Suki. Our thinking was if the boys saw I was capable of sending a text message, this would reassure them.

Antisocial I am not but I didn't mind being alone; it would have been difficult for me to talk anyway. One useful thing was that the side room had its own toilet facilities. I couldn't resist using them independently. I couldn't walk or even stand unsupported but there were plenty of hand holds in the small side ward. Every trip of a few yards to the loo was like a mountaineering adventure.

I am convinced that this unorthodox form of physiotherapy was of benefit to me, but it earned me reprimands from the staff. Next day, reading my hospital notes, I saw a black mark had been added to them about my unaided expeditions. It was as if I'd been given a written warning!

## [18] The Impatient Patient

The side ward detained me for only one day and one night. Afterwards, I had a whole large section, designed for a dozen patients, to myself. At least, I had it to myself for half-an-hour. At the end of this pleasant interlude eleven patients, wheeled in on their beds, started to arrive.

What had happened was that some senior person in the neurosurgical ward had decided to re-open a unit for we less dependent patients. I was glad to be able to count myself among their number. More especially, I felt it to be increasingly unlikely anyone was going to perform any neurosurgery upon me. My fear had been that someone might take the wrong bit out.

On my first morning I had two pieces of good news. The first was delivered by the friendly consultant (his name was John; I forget the surname) when he made his tour of inspection in company with a gaggle of lesser medical lights. He confirmed I was to have no 'medical intervention', was to be transferred to my local hospital as soon as a bed could be confirmed as being available and until then (here he addressed directly those that must have been the appropriate staff among his followers) I would receive excellent nursing care.

The second piece of good news was in my hospital notes, which naturally I looked at in more detail as soon as I was alone. These were largely couched in medical terms, naturally. No training was necessary for me to understand the significance of the sentence saying I was 'neurologically intact'. It was indeed the way I felt, even if still I couldn't stand unaided, let alone walk.

The only way I can think of my disconcerting state then is that trying to stand was like balancing one-legged on the top platform of a thirty-foot stepladder whilst trying to practise ballet points. Still, I did know that the cerebellum was the centre of balance and the bleeding had affected this area of my brain. I was simply going to have to be patient. What was more difficult to accept was my scrambled speech. I'd been here before.

This was reinforced when, on my first day in the new unit a friend of mine, Jack, rang on my mobile phone to ask why he hadn't heard from me for a week or so. He was shocked to hear me talk and could hardly understand a word I said. I thought I'd better send him a text message straight after our conversation, asking him to ring my home for information.

My problems with speech didn't stop me trying to hold long conversations with the nursing staff. The fact that much of my own side of these conversations must have been no more than semi-intelligible to them is more of a tribute to their patience and careful listening than the quality of my speech.

I remember leaning against the windowsill (leaning was essential) while one young nurse unburdened herself of some life-changing decisions lying before her. Meanwhile, the first heavy snow of winter was starting to fall outside. I suppose she spoke freely because I was a good listener. In fact, I must have been the ideal listener: a man who couldn't easily answer back.

More seriously, I can only speak in the highest terms of the nursing staff of all grades with whom I came into contact. With the increasing emphasis on what I would think of as the more technical side of nursing, at the expense of the old-style bedside nursing, we have surely lost a great deal. Personally, I was well enough to ensure (good-humouredly, I hope) that I received the attention I needed, but this wouldn't be true for all patients.

Mobility was something I needed a lot of help with. My independent motion was confined to the few feet around the bed I still found necessary for support. Even getting as far as the window was an achievement. To relieve myself was a real trek. I was unhappy at the prospect of using the bed-bottle I was offered.

Fortunately, the physiotherapists had advised the nursing staff that I would need to be supported by a nurse on each side to go to the toilet. In an odd way, these walks came to be one of the highlights of my day. I almost came to look forward to the sensation of my bladder filling. I made a point of joking with the staff on these little journeys so they wouldn't see them purely as a chore. Also, I wanted to try to keep up my own spirits.

After a couple of days, the physiotherapist told me I'd now need the precautionary support of only one nurse to walk to the toilet. Progress indeed. As I've said before, everything is relative.

The highlight of my days was naturally the evening visit from Suki. It was quite a distance from our home, and I was glad when she was able to travel with friends rather than on her own. Even then, I couldn't help feeling guilty about the journeys, often in adverse weather, they needed to make. The tail end of November, 2010 was very cold, with frequent snowfalls.

Most of my day was inevitably solitary. I did a lot of reading, but it's not possible to spend the whole day doing this, even when one is in the best of health. At least I didn't need to resort to the pay televisions once attached to the bed, as I did after my first 'episode' in the year 2000. These machines are now fortunately in the past. I'm sure they were only popular with hospitals, and then only for a for a short time, because they generated revenue. It was infuriatingly necessary to feed in quite significant amounts to get an hour's viewing of Freeview channels on the tiny screen.

There were three physiotherapists attached to the ward (I think they had other duties elsewhere, too). After a few days, the senior, a young lady called Becky, came to talk to me. She provided me with some notes on speech therapy, then explained that she was actually an occupational therapist. I was aghast. To me, this conjured up visions of a life of basket-making lying ahead of me. Fortunately, Becky quickly explained this wouldn't be the case; the physiotherapists would merely come to provide help with everyday mobility and living.

That's what happened. Soon I came to look forward to their visits. I went on long walks with some of them, or what seemed to me to be long walks, around the hospital. I performed tasks like picking things up from the floor, climbing a few of the stone steps and turning my head as far to the left and right as I could. These might have been simple, everyday actions, but they needed a great deal of concentration on my part. This therapy was a vitally important part of my treatment. I thought it a great pity that the therapists had to spend so much of their day writing notes rather than helping patients.

And I had an extra motivation to make progress. The day after Becky spoke to me, the staff nurse came to tell me there were no beds available at my local hospital. For the time being they'd arrange to transfer me to one of their own non-specialist wards. I reasoned that, if I didn't need treatment, I'd far sooner go home than be dumped in some forgotten corner of the hospital.

From that point on I waged a campaign for my discharge. The staff nurses who were responsible for the running of the unit bore the brunt of my nagging, but I also made sure the senior medical staff got the message on their ward rounds. I tried to do it all with a smile; I did not want to follow the example of one of the other patients whose bluff was called when he threatened to discharge himself. More importantly, I wanted to keep the staff on my side. I think I succeeded in this.

In the early afternoon of Wednesday, 1st December, 2010, I was talking to Amy, a young student nurse who had been working on the previous night shift and had been good enough to call in to see me for a chat before her afternoon shift began. Then the staff nurse for the unit came out to speak to me. Unexpectedly, she told me I was to be discharged and sent home by volunteer car as soon as my wife could be contacted.

Spontaneously, the two nurses broke into a dance of celebration. The other patients on the ward must have been wondering what was happening. I think the two were sharing my delight rather than celebrating their pleasure at being rid of me. At least, I hoped they were. I'd have joined them in their dance if only I'd been able to do it.

# The Longer Road Back

## [19] A Deep and Dark December

I was delighted to see Suki's arrival an hour or so after what I will always think of the nurses' dance celebrating my escape. She'd had to travel from our home by public transport.

From the neurosurgical ward a friendly porter, the same one who'd taken me down to have a brain scan a week or so before, wheeled me the longer distance to what they called 'The Pre-discharge Suite'. Suki walked with us.

This was promising. I liked the name of the place where I was heading. It turned out to be nothing more than a medium-size room with a television in the corner, plus two cheerful members of staff who periodically waved my fellow escapees goodbye. There seemed to be a large number of them, most ahead of me in the queue. For what seemed like hours, but was assuredly nothing of the kind, I sat dumbly in the chair, wondering when my turn would come. I tried to read a few of the magazines but what I have always thought of as waiting room torpor took over. It prevented my mind from absorbing anything I tried to read, even the captions below the pictures.

Eventually, the driver came. He was an ordinary member of the public paid, so he told me, a volunteer mileage rate to take home discharged patients who required transport, though who didn't need an ambulance. I was glad to be in this category myself. Nevertheless, I was grateful for his support to walk from the discharge lounge to his car.

I sat in the front passenger seat and gave him directions. These were simple: along the motorway and, after leaving it, across six roundabouts to take the right turn at the last. Easy as it was, I kept rehearsing the route in my mind and thinking about how to announce each step of it: I'd feel an idiot if I took us down a wrong turning. Fortunately, he understood me well enough and we stopped outside my house with no problem. He helped me to my front door and refused our offer of a cup of tea. This was it. I was home. I was an ex-patient.

*

It was the first day of a dark and far colder than normal December. Suki gave me a blanket to cover my legs and I sat in the chair. What should I do? The first thing I in fact did was switch on the computer to answer a few e-mails people had been good enough to send me. After this, I was pleased to renew my acquaintance with the radio, hi-fi, and a few books.

My life was confined to the chair at first. Before long I managed to stumble around the downstairs rooms with the help of handholds and even managed to go upstairs although, for safety reasons, I had to do this as a semi-climbing exercise with much planning and care. The return journey was even less dignified since I had to do it in reverse. Still, I was glad to be able to undertake this exotic expedition.

Later that afternoon, I had my first bath for a while. This took some doing. I couldn't climb into the bath unaided and I dared not sit down for fear of being unable to clamber out again. What we did was put a chair in the bath and then carefully manoeuvre me on to the seat. Suki was then able to sluice me down with jugs of water. It took a lot of time and effort on both of our parts, but it was worth it as far as I was concerned. I've never felt so clean in all my life.

I needed help to dress for the next three or four mornings. The simplest things like pulling on my socks were a challenge. If I had to visit the bathroom in the night the journey needed careful thought, with me making full use of the walls and every possible support. But each day I progressed. Little improvements like getting my own shirt over my head were important milestones.

A week or so before the holiday, Suki wanted to go to Cardiff to get some bits and pieces for Christmas. We asked our neighbours, Steve and June, both then in their eighties, to 'baby sit' for me and kept in touch with each other by text. Telephone calls were still beyond me, as indeed was a chat with Steve and June, much to their puzzlement and my frustration. June lent me one of her walking sticks. This was immensely helpful to me, but I was glad to be able to return it after three days' use.

Beside emails, I had half-a-dozen or so personal visitors in the earlier part of the month. This cheered me up enormously, especially since much of the time there was a lot of snow about. Our next-door-neighbour, Debbie, came around one day. She slipped over on the drive, fracturing both her wrists. Plaster casts were not the Christmas decorations she'd planned on having.

I was not to leave the house and its environs for the rest of the month. In fact, the first time I ventured out was on 4th January, when I travelled the two miles to the local hospital for a CT scan of my brain. This was the third such scan I'd had in five or six weeks. I was to have another a month or two later. I was beginning to get worried about having my brain fried by all this attention. More seriously, I was pleased that the scan on 4th January and the subsequent one showed a big improvement since late November.

Before that, the month of December wore on. I was improving day by day, if not as quickly as I'd have liked. Mind you, I have to admit I wouldn't have been satisfied unless the fairy flew down from our Christmas tree, waved her magic wand and said, 'It's all right. You can wake up now.'

## [20] Physiotherapy

While I was still in The Heath Hospital, the Occupational Therapist, Becky, had told me she'd be referring me to an organisation grandly named the 'Community Integrated Intermediate Care Service'. The 'Reablement Team' would be able to help me with physiotherapy as well as speech and language therapy. I knew I was in serious need of both.

The names may be peculiar, but the help the service gave me was invaluable. I do hope it is not to fall victim to public spending cuts and that others will continue to be able to benefit as I did. The last time I checked they were surviving, but it doesn't need much imagination to see they'd make a soft target for miscalled 'efficiency savings'.

Not long after my discharge from hospital on 1st December, a senior from the team, whose name I think was Fiona, came to see me. I suppose the official reason for her visit was to assess what help I'd need, but I must record that her manner was informal and friendly.

Naturally, we talked about the problems I had with locomotion and other simple physical actions. I explained that, although I still found it difficult to walk steadily without the use of frequent hand-holds, or even stand for more than a second or two, I could ascend and descend the stairs, provided I did so on all fours; in reverse when coming down. This was as well: our only lavatory is upstairs.

Fiona arranged for a handrail to be fitted on the wall adjacent to the stairs, to replace the half-length one fitted by our neighbour, Peter, ten years before. There was also to be a new, shorter one at the top of our stairs where the existing banister ended. I still make use of them, though am pleased now to record I am only really dependent upon them for making a safe descent of the stairs with my double vision. I don't any longer have to rely on them to hoist myself up.

She also arranged for the delivery of a commode and some sort of support structure to put across the bath. It was a relief to me when I didn't have to use either. Fiona also told me the physiotherapist would be arriving soon, although I wouldn't be seeing the speech therapist until January.

The first physiotherapist to call we knew as 'Bobby', which was the name he preferred to use in his work. I suppose this was to make life easier for his 'clients', who might have had difficulty with his given Indian name. He came along with a young student therapist. I'm afraid I can't recall her name, but she lived in Aberdare, about 25 miles north of my home. On this first visit, they wanted me to use the stairs, go through a few more 'everyday' actions and to a play a catching game with my granddaughter's beach ball. The last was silly fun in its way, even though I had to explain that my greatest difficulty was supplied by the double vision I'd lived with for the last ten years.

One day not long after this first visit, we awoke to the sight of thick snow on the ground. Snow was still falling. No traffic was moving. Bobby was due to arrive, I think for only my second appointment, on that morning. We knew he lived about two miles away so didn't think it at all likely that he'd be able to make it. We went back to bed.

About twenty minutes later there came an insistent knocking on the door. I volunteered to go down to see who it could be. When I opened the door, I saw a man standing in the snow before me. He was wrapped in a voluminous scarf over a thick coat and wore a white woollen cap, pulled down over his ears. I didn't recognise him.

'Yes?' I thought he must be the driver of a car that had broken down in the harsh conditions. What on Earth was he doing out on the road on a day like this?

'It's Bobby,' he said.

Bobby had walked all the way to my house. He explained that the policy of his team was to call at the homes of clients, to make sure we didn't need any 'emergency supplies'. He asked if we had enough bread and milk. Emergency milk is a concept I've never personally understood. Bread I could understand, though not milk. But I do know that many people would rate milky tea above even bread in importance. I had the good grace to keep this observation to myself. Suki was downstairs by this time and together we explained we were fine.

Bobby asked if we could give him directions to a nearby road where lived another client of his. I was able to lend him a local street atlas. Then he said he wanted to give me a physiotherapy session before he left. I said this wouldn't be necessary on such a morning; he should go on and do what he had to do elsewhere. To be honest, I was thinking as much as anything about the fact that I hadn't yet had breakfast.

'Oh, come on, man! I've come all this way through the snow and now you say you don't want therapy?' he protested. So, shamefacedly, and breakfastless, I had my therapy session on that day after all.

The unusual combination of a Christmas visit to Delhi and New Year celebrations in Trafalgar square called to Bobby over the holiday period so another member of the team, Eunice, deputised for three visits. She came once before and twice after Christmas – she went away for Christmas itself for a family visit to Pembroke. Eunice was a bit of a character, always laughing and joking.

She gave me the scheduled physiotherapy exercises but, when she saw I was making good progress, she was happy to start me on my way with speech therapy. She said this wasn't her area of expertise but volunteered to go through the printed exercises given to me by Becky in The Heath Hospital. We both had a lot of fun going through the 'oos', 'ees' and 'buh', 'puh' and 'muh' sounds.

Bobby returned twice more to give me exercises in January. On the second of these visits we walked fifty yards or so down and up the hill on my road. I felt the effort of ascending the incline more than I was used to doing on the return, uphill leg of the journey. But Bobby was highly satisfied. When we got back indoors, he told Suki he was pleased with my progress and she could now take me out for short walks. We didn't like to tell him she'd already been doing this for a couple of days!

Fiona called for a brief 'signing off' visit on 12th January. The next day Eunice called for my final physiotherapy session. On the day after that, Bobby called in, simply to say goodbye. It was a pleasant way to end this part of my treatment.

That same Friday evening, with the help of my friend Joyce, I attended a meeting of our local writers' group, of which I was then still a member. I ventured out three times more in January. Two of these were to make visits to our local hospital. The first occasion was to have another CAT ('computerised tomography') scan of my brain and on the second I had my first out-patient appointment with a doctor.

The other time I went out was to attend a meeting of a more informal discussion group called 'The 05'. I wasn't capable of much in the way of discussion, but these were the first times since earlier in the previous November I'd been able to attend either group. It was good to be back in circulation again.

## [21] Bonjour to a White Christmas

The wintry conditions beginning while I was in hospital in later November had continued until the early part of the next month, with sporadic but heavy snowfalls. For a few days the snow cleared but then it returned around the middle of the December. I don't think 2010 was technically a 'White Christmas', in that no snow fell after Christmas Eve. The bookies wouldn't have paid out a penny on it, but certainly there were still heavy drifts of snow on the ground until after Christmas Day.

I wasn't around for the winter of 1946/47, when the Government found it necessary to draw-up emergency famine plans, though certainly remember the freezing temperatures of the winters of 1962/1963 and 1981/82. There were even a few brief flurries of snow one Christmas day a few years earlier in this Millennium. For me, though, 2010/11 is the winter in my mind as being the one with the 'White Christmas'.

Edmund was due to arrive with my daughter-in-law, Ping, and my granddaughter, Annabella, early on the evening of Monday 20th, the start of the week before Christmas. They were travelling by train from Portsmouth, a trundling cross-country journey. They were lucky enough to find a half-open window of opportunity to travel through the freezing conditions and arrived less than an hour late.

My granddaughter Annabella, aged a few months over two at the time, was puzzled to find me in a chair with a blanket over my legs. I was still unable to stand or walk steadily at this point. She was even more puzzled when she spoke to me. At the time, she was truly bilingual, having been born in Shanghai. When she couldn't understand my response to her greeting, she tried again in Mandarin. When she still couldn't understand my response, she said, very clearly and loudly, 'BONJOUR!'

Suki and I had jokingly taught her a few French expressions months before. Later, during the next year, she said to Suki, 'Nanna, why does Grandpa speak a funny language?'

Only fairly recently has she started to come to terms with the fact that her grandfather can't speak properly.

It was strange for Edmund to find himself having to help me in and out of the bath. I was glad when, before his return to Portsmouth, I was able to do it with only the aid of the short bath rail fitted by Peter ten years before.

Edmund was pressed into service wielding a shovel to clear the path. Suki and Ping helped him. I couldn't lend a hand but was pleased to find myself able to stumble out to retrieve Annabella, who had taken advantage of all the adult activity to wander up toward our garden pond. In all probability, the ice would have been thick enough to support her, but we were glad we didn't have to find out.

Joseph could only be with us for a short time that Christmas because of work demands: he was temporarily undertaking two part-time jobs in London at the time. He didn't arrive until fairly late on Christmas Eve and had to return early on the Monday following Boxing Day. More snow had fallen not long before his visit and we anxiously kept in touch with him during his train journey. Fortunately, he arrived from Paddington not too late, although some trains were cancelled following a fire in the London terminal. The rest were incredibly crowded. My sister Mary also came to us on Christmas Eve. Fortunately, she lives only a mile away and had no travel difficulties.

So, we were able to have a family Christmas, despite all the obstacles thrown in our way. I wasn't able to express myself at all well but was grateful for the day and all that it meant. We go in for the traditional Christmas Dinner, with roast turkey, plum-pudding and crackers. This is something Suki and I appreciate every year, but the food tasted especially good in 2010. For the first year, Joseph was responsible for making the white sauce for the pudding, under instruction from his Aunt Mary.

After Christmas, when Joseph's flying visit had come to an end, Edmund and Annabella and, to a lesser extent, Ping, all came down with viral infections. Annabella had to be taken to our doctor's surgery for a prescription. Thankfully, the minor health problems all cleared up in short order. It was odd, though definitely rewarding, to be able to provide a small share of the nursing care.

On 30th December, it was time for Edmund and his family to return to Portsmouth. They took a taxi to the railway station. I was pleased to be able to walk out, unaided, to the pavement in front of the house to wave them off. Small steps indeed, but this was an important sign to me that I was on the road to recovery.

## [22] Weighty Matters

At the beginning of the Millennium year I weighed well over fourteen-and-a-half stone (93kg). I am not slightly built, so this wasn't anything like grossly obese. It was, though, more weight than, ideally, I should have been carrying. When I came out of hospital after my three-week stay on 11th April, I was down to under eleven-and-a-half stones (72kg).

I ate next to nothing for my first week as an in-patient and had a small appetite for the next two. This is not a comment on the hospital food!

Having lost so much weight so drastically, I resolved to keep most of it off. I decided that around twelve to twelve-and-a-half stones (76kg to 80kg) should be about right for me. My difficulty was I liked food and drink and soon found my appetite returning. I wasn't interested in a quick fix crash diet; I'd already had that. I was in it for the long term.

The only thing for it was to watch my intake along with ensuring I had regular exercise. Fortunately, I've never been one for snacks and sweets or eating between meals, even when I was a child. These have never been among my sins. I thought all I'd have to do was fix a big 'NO!' sign in my mind and keep to regular, small meals. It wasn't to be quite this simple in practice.

I didn't do too badly, but it was always a struggle. Over the next ten years, before my 'second episode', my weight had crept up to nearer thirteen stones rather than my target maximum of twelve-and-a-half. My stay in hospital was only of a week's duration this time and no unconsciousness was involved, but it did bring my weight down to slightly below the upper limit I'd fixed. Still, this wasn't the way I wanted to do it. A more sensible course of action was needed.

What I did was generally keep to a strict diet as before, but with a difference. My plan was to have a bowl of cereal or porridge and toast for breakfast. This would be followed by a lunch consisting of a yoghurt drink with plant stenol and three fruits with a pint of water. Sometimes I'd add a wheat biscuit to this feast. I'd keep to my saintly ways by having a not-too-large evening meal with plenty of vegetables and a restricted quantity of meat. Naturally, I thought it wise to drink plenty of water at other times. Does this sound boring? It was. It's the sort of thing you'd read in a hectoring magazine article.

The difference now is that if I fancy something less healthy – say a large steak, one of those delicious (but very fatty) pork pies or a glass or two extra of beer or wine – I have it. It's something I know I can't do too often. I weigh myself at least weekly to find out where I am on my personally permitted weight range. This became 11 stones 10 pounds and 12 stones 3 pounds – it's a few pounds lower now. If I find myself edging toward the higher end of the scale, I know I need to postpone the pork pies for a week or fortnight. If I have a large lunch, I know I have to make amends with a minimalist evening meal.

As we get older, we need less food. It's largely a matter of modifying eating habits. Over time you don't miss big meals half as much.

'Episode two' did bring me an unlooked-for aid in my continued efforts towards weight control. The damage then made to my swallowing reflex (this didn't happen in the year 2000) now means I have to make a conscious effort to chew every mouthful. I make a point of telling people that I can't talk when I'm eating. They usually answer 'none of us should' but I tell them I really can't do it. This has nothing to do with manners in my case. Having to eat slowly and carefully does have a plus side. It means that I can actually enjoy the taste of the food more, so need less of it.

If I'd have been truly aware of a simple thing like this years ago, I'd have determined to eat more slowly long before now!

## [23] Minor Matters

I've said a lot about the more significant problems that have affected me since the Millennium Year. Most of the initial problems, though serious in 2000 and 2010 and the years immediately after, have been overcome pleasingly quickly.

My dexterity has recovered to a large degree, though very slowly. For safety originally, and because I've now acquired the habit, I still shave with my left hand and far prefer to write with a keyboard than in freehand. In combination with my diplopia, my damaged hand co-ordination can cause me unexpected difficulties. Still, with patience and one eye closed or covered I can perform quite delicate manual tasks. I could never have claimed to be particularly adept with my hands, anyway.

I have accepted that double vision is now a permanent feature of my life and that I will be a 'work in progress' with being able to use reasonable speech for some time yet to come (I hope it is 'still yet to come').

What about the rest? Well, I am now some years older than I was when my life changed at the Millennium, so don't expect to be entering any marathon races, to climb Kilimanjaro or win any dancing competitions. The majority of people of my age or even a fair bit younger don't do these things, anyway. I have to concern myself with the more modest things that constitute 'normal' living.

To be perfectly honest, I have little cause for complaint. There are only a few additional things I have to think hard about.

One of these minor issues that puzzles me slightly is my diminished sense of direction. Of course, this isn't a true 'sense' at all. But some people seem to have the instincts of a homing pigeon. I was never one of them, although can at least lay claim to have written a walking book in the early nineties. For this, I needed to design, test (i.e. walk!) and draw the initial route maps as well as writing the route directions and similar things. I'd have great difficulty in repeating some of this now.

I've never been able to decide for myself how much of the problem is caused by my double vision. Obviously, it doesn't help (particularly indoors, where distances are shorter) but it doesn't explain everything. At an early stage of my first recovery, I went for quite a long walk with my sons. At one point I wanted to take them in entirely the wrong direction – north instead of south – from a river bridge we all knew well. Since that day I have been careful to plan out every new route I take, even quite short ones within an unfamiliar building, rather than rely on 'instincts' to which I can no longer lay claim.

My second 'episode' in 2010 brought one new problem. My swallowing reflex was affected. The damage was only partial, thank goodness. Generally speaking, I have learned to cope with the problems it brings. In the Heath Hospital, I stayed quiet about it – my main objective then was to 'escape' as quickly as I could – and kept to a gentle diet, like preferring wheat biscuits and porridge to the more fibrous morning cereals.

It surprised me when I was home to find breakfast to be the most challenging meal of the day. Perhaps this is because my senses are not fully alert early in the morning. More likely it is the combination of solid cereal and liquid drink presenting the difficulty. At all events, I spluttered through the first dozen or so breakfasts. But I persevered and, as the weeks passed, found I was choking more rarely.

Even now, though, I have to very consciously 'shape' my throat as I take each mouthful. If I even *think* of talking at these times (this is not hyperbole) woe betide me. I tell new dining companions I can't talk when I'm eating. The invariable reply is 'none of us should. It's not good manners.'

Maybe, but in practice everyone talks when they're eating, even if they don't do it with their mouths full. Mealtimes would be poorer without a bit of conversation. 'Good manners' are forced upon me when my mouth is full. By the time I finish a mouthful the time has often passed for me to say what I was going to say!

Still, there are benefits: now I really taste every mouthful of food. As for wine and beer, these are things I've always liked. But now I *really* like them!

I've been fortunate in that I've had few side-effects from the medication prescribed for me. After my first illness this was light enough: now I have only a single 5mg dose of Amlodipine and a single 25mg dose of Atenolol. The original dosages were halved in 2000 and then halved again in 2001. Neither was increased in 2010, when I had my 'second episode', I'm pleased to say. In fact, the only side-effect I have from one or both (I don't know which) of them is feeling of chill actually inside in my right-side lower limb extremities. In plainer language, I often have a cold right hand or foot. This is something I can experience even on warm days. Still, I know the medication is something with which it is sensible to persevere.

I've been lucky enough not to have to take too many drugs throughout my life and therefore have had few side-effects. The only one I recall in the last century was in 1977, when I experienced a violent stomach reaction to an iron tablet. This was something our Blood Donation Centre prescribed routinely in those days. In the morning I could hardly move. I probably wouldn't have stirred out of bed if I didn't have an important job interview coming up that day. Somehow, I got through it and ended up with the job.

The only side-effect I've experienced in our present century was to Simvastatin, the anti-cholesterol tablets, prescribed for me in about 2004. My cholesterol level has never been high, although was above the NHS target level. The tablets gave me extreme discomfort in my right calf muscle. I could hardly walk. I spoke to my then general practitioner, Dr Mohajer. She suggested I should stop the tablets and instead try taking a daily drink containing plant stenol extracts. These are widely available in supermarkets and elsewhere.

Before his retirement a few years ago, I had a long conversation with our senior GP, Dr Lodwick on this subject. He wasn't a fan of stenol drinks. His line was 'if you want to spend your money, go ahead and buy them. But your blood pressure and cholesterol levels are fine, so I'm not going to recommend Simvastatins, either'.

I thought about what he'd said but decided to continue with a stenol drink every day. I treat it as part of my medication. I'm pleased to report that this has been successful in controlling and even reducing the level of cholesterol in my blood. And they are far tastier than those Simvastatin tablets!

## [24] Speech Therapy

Soon after arriving at our home for the first time on 10th January, 2011, Stephanie Godfrey, my assigned speech therapist, made what was clearly her prepared introductory statement of the afternoon. Stephanie was an experienced practitioner and must have said a similar thing many times before.

'Am I to call you Mr East?' she said. 'Or would you prefer it if I called you Tom?'

'You can call me Sir if you like,' I replied (not expressed perfectly, I should say). 'But if you do that, I'm going to call you Madam.'

For a moment she was startled. I think she might have contemplated running screaming from the house. Then, fortunately, she realised I was teasing. It broke the ice, and everything went easily after that. This was the first and last standard gambit she offered to me, I'm sure. Suki was present for all six of our sessions. She took a full part in all the conversations and she and Stephanie got on well.

I found the six weeks of therapy highly beneficial. It might have been on the dull side to read out lists of words and syllable sounds but for me, less than two months after my second haemorrhage, it was a major challenge.

The various tips she passed on, like the key role in speech played by the simple process of breathing, the need to prepare for speaking and the extra importance of correct posture when one has other difficulties to deal with were immediately useful to me and have been since. Appendix 4 (page 149) is the actual 'script' I typed one day to record on her telephone voicemail. Appendix 8 (page 157) reproduces the 'speech card' Stephanie gave me, plus the later copy of it made for me in Malaysia by my brother-in-law Wai Fan.

But the six weeks came to an end. Almost the last thing Stephanie said to me was 'you've got the tool kit. Don't be afraid to give yourself speech therapy sessions.' Yes, I had the tool kit, but not yet the ability to use it effectively. Reading lists of words and simple passages to myself became increasingly dull and I wasn't yet ready to read more interesting things aloud or to embark on anything more adventurous.

What I did was to try my best to carry on as normal with groups of people. My speech was far from normal, of course, but I am grateful to the many who put up with my earliest struggles.

In February or March, 2001, for instance, I gave a joint talk to our local writers' group with another member, Kay. What 'joint' meant in practice was that I wrote everything down and Kay presented it, trying not to make it look too much as if she were reading from a script. She did well in this aim, I should say. The fact that we designed the session to encourage audience participation helped things along, I'm sure.

I also attended a smaller more informal, writing group, originally named '05' (so called because it had been initiated in 2005). This is aimed at critiques of manuscripts and useful for this purpose it has been. The other members, at various times, have been Carol, Chris, Dominique, Jan, Jean, Pat and Rowland. With the cooperation and tolerance of my friends, for a period of about three months, we added a half-time 'speech-therapy interlude.'

In this, I read aloud short passages I'd written, while they did their best to make notes of what I was saying. Afterwards, I quizzed them about the details of what I'd read, all the time trying to stress that I was 'marking' myself and not them. Still, it was tougher on the listeners than me, especially since one had hearing problems and another was unused to the disciplines of note taking. All the benefits came to me from this exercise, I have to admit. I subsequently used the short notes I'd read from as the basis for a longer piece of writing, *A Fifties Childhood*.

Another thing I did was resume my attendance at a poetry group. We called it 'Poems and Pints'. One purpose of the group was to read poems aloud, both those by the reader and those written by well-known poets. As you'll probably guess from the name, the other main purpose is to consume pints or their equivalent. The effort of reading aloud and trying to make myself intelligible to an audience was useful to me, although I'm not sure how much people could follow, particularly the early days.

Naturally, I also tried to play my part in normal group conversations, something I'd largely regained the ability to do before my 'second episode' shook me out of my complacency. 'Group' here means anything upwards of three people.

A thing I'd barely noticed before my difficulties is that there is an element of what I have come to think of as 'competitive talking' in any group conversation. This is especially true where people have a lot they want to say. This is often the case with my friends! In order to get their voices and opinions heard, people often interrupt each other, crosstalk and unconsciously use the various techniques and tricks of conversation and debate.

It is interesting to watch this in a dispassionate way and there is absolutely nothing rude or impolite about the process. These are merely the normal mechanics of human conversation at work. The trouble for me is, when I want to say anything, I do it so ponderously that, in a sense, the world has to stop while I speak. I am grateful to the many people who allow the world to cease its motion while I have my say.

Some two-and-a-half-years after my 'second episode', I became increasingly aware that my progress towards normal speech was alarmingly slow. My joking calculation, surely not far off the truth, was that, at my present rate of progress, I should be word-perfect by the time I was 165 years old!

The slow progress shouldn't have surprised me; after all I was now trying to find my second set of alternate neural pathways. I knew I was making *some* progress. My sister-in-law Wanda from Australia, remarked in 2012 that I could now walk and talk at the same time, something I hadn't been able to do when she'd seen me in the UK a year before. Still, I was hoping for something a bit quicker!

What I decided to do eventually was to start to give myself semi-formal speech therapy sessions, exactly as Stephanie had recommended some time before. I gave a lot of thought to this and decided on the following pattern:

1. Reading a poem of my own.
2. Reading a poem by someone else.
3. Singing a song.
4. Walking up and down stairs eight times, counting the numbers one to twelve in various languages.

With the addition of a few simple physical exercises designed to maintain my arm strength – essential when coming downstairs with double vision – it all takes about twenty to twenty-five minutes each morning. I could count the number of sessions I've missed (for example, when I've needed to leave home early) on the fingers of one hand. Otherwise, I try to do the whole thing 365 days a year and to start with made it a point of honour to complete the task before I touched breakfast. To avoid being acutely bored by the process, I vary my choices in 1-3, on a roughly fortnightly cycle.

The language pattern I follow is 1 – Breton, 2 – Cantonese, 3 – Romanian, 4 – German, 5 – Malay, 6 – French, 7 – Spanish, 8 – Welsh. At the present time I'm trying to motivate myself to add Mandarin and Latin rounds.

If this list sounds impressive let me be strictly honest and say that in some of these languages, I can't do much more than count to twelve, say please or thank you and ask for a beer or coffee. In some of them I can't even do this much.

The idea for 'stair-counting' came from an exercise Stephanie had me doing towards the end of the six weeks she helped me. With this 'prototype' there were only two 'rounds' and both were in English. My thought was that repeating the exercise eight times rather than twice should aid my breath control. Forcing myself to speak in different languages should not only tax my powers of enunciation (the Romanian for 'eleven' is 'unsprezece'; still not so easy to say when you're on the eleventh step up and have aphasia) but also make me think at the same time. This seems to work: if my concentration lapses, I can easily find myself starting to count, say, in Spanish and switching unconsciously to Romanian, in which the some of the numbers start with similar sounds.

In 2014 I expressed all this as a poem, *Speech Therapy, Part One*. This is reproduced as appendix 6 (page 153). It reflects the situation exactly as I saw it. Apart from the first line, section 1 does in fact incorporate one of the first poems I read when I returned to our local 'poems and pints group'. The word 'pause' is read aloud – followed by a lengthy pause!

The song lines in the poem are intended to be sung. The example I have used in appendix 6 is a non-copyright, traditional ballad that comes in numerous versions. However, my favourite is a more recent song of West Indian origin. When it comes to the turn of *Fat Man* to be part of my morning therapy, this is a song I always sing in full, and at the highest volume I can manage. My version doesn't bear much relation to the that by Desmond Dekker but I'm sure it helps me. And it's always good fun. It used to send my granddaughter, Annabella, into fits of the giggles when she was younger. I'm grateful to the songwriter, Derrick Seymour Morgan.

I see the footnote as an integral part of the poem. Indeed, it was some of this that gave me the idea to write it in the first place. The note is made up from part of an actual email sent to me by my friend Chris and my genuine reaction to it. Each time I have read the poem I've had someone else (it can't be me, because of its content) read the footnote before I read the poem.

The brief second section is a more or less direct quotation of Stephanie's words and my initial thoughts when I heard them, and for a long time afterward. The 'now' final section describes, in abbreviated form, the actual pattern of my morning exercises. Naturally, I read this poem at the 'poems and pints' group a couple of years after I resumed attendance – as soon as I'd written it, in fact.

I also read it at a bigger group in Neath, to the west of where I live. I returned to this one a few years after I went back to my local group. This meant I didn't know all of those present. It pleases me that I soon got to know most of the people and a number of them have been brave enough to read with me. Step forward, Alan, Bee, Liza and Wes.

My biggest tests came in Cardiff in 2014 and Llanelli in 2015. *Speech Therapy, Part 1* was the poem I chose to read in front of around fifty or sixty people on each occasion, many of whom were not known to me. I'm glad to say the readings were well received. I think of this poem as custom-built for me. Few other people would be able to read it in quite the authentic way I do!

I had something of a surprise after my Cardiff performance, though. One of the people in the audience turned out to be a Romanian lady. Georgeta did tell me that my pronunciation of 'un, doi, trei' ('one, two, three') was fine. I hope she wasn't merely being polite. She would certainly have been generous if the poem had counted all the way up to twelve. 'Six' and 'seven' ('şase' and 'şapte' in Romanian) begin with a 'sh' sound, a combination of letters that even now sometimes gives me trouble.

In 2017 I felt bold enough to add *Speech Therapy, Part 2* to this. The two poems are given as appendices 5 and 6, pp 153 to 153. I have no immediate plans to put a part 3 together!

So, where is my speech now? I have to think of myself as not yet far enough from my departure point. I'm still limping along the road. But at least I'm limping slightly faster these days.

## [25] Investigations

In early 2011, I went for my post-admission consultation at my local hospital. I didn't at first see the consultant, but a polite young registrar whose name I regret I've forgotten. He asked how I was, and in the peculiar speech I had at the time (far more peculiar than it is now) I answered him. Then he asked how my mobility was coming along.

'I can get up from this chair without using my arms,' I said. He was surprised. I hadn't been out of hospital for much more than a month.

'Go on, then,' he said. 'Show me.'

This I did, hoping I wouldn't fall over. He was impressed and immediately went to see the senior consultant, Dr Mukhopadhyay. A pleasant, friendly man, the consultant came in to talk to me. After our conversation, he told his registrar to arrange a series of tests. The registrar blanched at the list of investigations.

As did I. These were an echocardiogram (heart scan), a 24-hour ambulatory monitoring of my blood pressure, a repeat brain scan, urinary tests for cortisol, normetadrenaline and metadrenaline. There was a blood scan to measure kidney function, liver function, bone profile, thyroid function, folic acid levels, Vitamin B12 and ferritin levels, clotting and normal blood counts.

Of these, I remember the blood pressure monitoring, the heart scan and the brain scan best. I think this was the order in which I had them. They all came quite quickly. I think also the registrar arranged for them in the order I have given. I know for sure that the blood pressure monitoring took place on 28th February/1st March, 2011 because, just in case something untoward should be discovered, I made a record of my activities during the monitoring. This is given as Appendix 9 (page 159, should you wish to glance at it. Not that my activities on that day and night had much zing about them, you'll understand.

What 'ambulatory' means in this sense is that the lucky person is fitted with a quite hefty (there are, no doubt, lighter devices around today) piece of equipment  which continuously monitors blood pressure through the normal span of a day and night. While doing things like going on the bus, watching a bit of TV and so on, the monitor is doing its stuff. I have to say I felt like a rather clunky prototype robot whilst it was going on.

In fact, while I was being monitored, I found the night hardest to cope with. When I record in the appendix that at such-and-such time I was 'awoken by monitor activity' this is something of an understatement. A more accurate rendition would have been 'monitor invaded my dreams'.

The feeling was weird in the extreme. Still, I knew that the purpose of the test might be of benefit to me and both times I was awoken I was able to get back to sleep without too much difficulty. Nevertheless, I was relieved to be able to disengage with the monitor next morning after breakfast.

I had to attend hospital for the heart scan. This is the only occasion on which my heart has been checked, other than routinely with a stethoscope. This experience was also peculiar. There wasn't really anything so odd in a physical sense, where all that happens is that the monitoring device is slid around or held against the chest and back. This does seem to go on for quite some time, but it is the strangest thing was to be watching the image of my heart on the screen. I couldn't take my eyes off the image glooping noisily around at my side.

To settle me down, or perhaps simply because she was a friendly person, the technician talked to me the whole time. I found out that she was from South America and shared the name of our granddaughter, Annabella. My heart seemed to be going through alarming antics on the screen, so I was pleased when, at the conclusion of the test, Annabella told me my heart was very sound.

The brain scan was the least pleasant of the experiences. This wasn't the first I've had: it was my fourth since the previous

23rd November. I'd had one when I was first admitted to the A&E unit of my local hospital, one a few days after I was transferred to the neurosurgical ward of the Heath Hospital and a third at my local hospital in early January.

This time, I had to drink a small quantity of purplish liquid beforehand. I was told that the purpose of this was to enhance the quality of the scanned image. I was also told it would make me feel warm for a moment. This it certainly did. As I have said elsewhere, going into a monitor is not an experience to savour. Going in whilst feeling suddenly flushed all over doesn't improve the experience. Still, I have to admit the warm feeling only lasts for a minute or two. Menopausal women, who get no notice of when flushes will occur, my heart goes out to you.

When all the tests were completed by April, 2011, Dr Mukhopadhyay wrote me a helpful and explicatory letter giving me details of the test results. Never have I been so pleased to read the word 'normal' repeated quite as often. He also told me my average blood pressure over the hours of monitoring was 111/68, which in fact is slightly on the low side. Most reassuringly to me, he informed me that the brain scan had revealed 'resolution of the haematoma'. In other words, there was no blood clot to be seen.

I wrote a brief 'thank you' letter in response to this. In fact, I took the opportunity to deliver it in person because I had an appointment booked with him only a day or two later. This hard-pressed NHS consultant took the trouble to ensure I'd understood everything he'd written in the letter. Then he told me that he could not explain why I'd had the haemorrhage in the first place, exactly as no explanation had been found for my 'episode one' in the Millennium Year.

He was probably a little surprised when I readily accepted this. But isn't it better to get the answer 'we don't know why' than something like 'you've got a dickie heart' or 'you have a clapped-out kidney?'

This point was reinforced by Dr Mukhopadhyay. 'If you give me your brain to examine on a bench,' he said jokingly. 'I'll probably be able to tell you more.'

'No thanks' I said. 'I'm still using it.'

We both laughed at our exchange. This part of our discussion may have been frivolous but there was a serious point behind it.

## [26] Learning Welsh

One of the consequences of my 'second episode' at the end of 2010 was that I had to abandon the Welsh language classes I'd started only the year before. I'd been some months late in enrolling, although was reasonably confident I'd be able to catch up. The teacher, Heledd Smith, was a helpful and pleasant young woman. Although her class was full and I could see she had some misgivings about taking me on, she gave me the nod with a smile.

My decision to apply for these morning classes had been prompted by the sight of a poster in the window of our local newsagent. The notice should probably have been taken down months before. I'm glad it wasn't.

In the event, I coped well enough. The pace was relaxed and undemanding. Although the majority of my fellow-students had studied Welsh at school level, in most cases their experience was anything between twenty and sixty years in the past, so this made no major difference. Anyway, I had previously studied some Welsh myself. On that occasion it was in evening classes. This was in the early nineteen-nineties. The teacher, a lively and enthusiastic young woman called Christine Jenkins, later became my sons' Welsh teacher in school. It was fun to tease them by saying we'd all had the same teacher.

In the nineteen-nineties, I worked in a busy job in Cardiff. Unfortunately, I often returned home too late to go to my evening classes. In all, I managed to attend fewer than three-quarters of them.

Nevertheless, I enjoyed those I could attend. As I did, my fellow-students responded well to Christine's approach. Her unfailing cheerfulness was some achievement considering she'd previously spent a day with pupils in the school where she worked at the time. Despite my sporadic attendance, I managed to complete the first year of the course and even started the second. Then I had to admit defeat: I knew I was likely to be able to attend only about half the sessions in the coming year. This wasn't enough, so I took the soft option and stopped trying.

When I picked up my studies again in 2009, I found that most of my fellow students were natives of Wales. I'd attended school in London where Welsh was not taught or used. This presented no great difficulty, though. Welsh was not a wholly unfamiliar language to me.

My father had been brought up as a Welsh-speaker. It was the speech used for everyday purposes in his childhood home. Indeed, my father's mother, although she died soon after his birth, was recorded as a monoglot Welsh speaker in the census. The stepmother who raised him also preferred to speak in Welsh, as did both of my grandfathers.

Although my father had largely left the language behind when he, with the rest of my family moved to London in 1936, my mother, not herself a fluent Welsh-speaker, had used it fairly indiscriminately with me in my pre-school years. When I did start infants' school, I was puzzled as to why the other children couldn't understand sentences like '*Mae hi'n bwrw glaw*' ('it's raining'). They, in turn, wondered why I called my mother 'Mam'.

My family was very conscious of its Welsh identity. My parents were both born and bred in the Rhondda Fach. The elder of my two brothers and my sister were also born in this valley. All three of my siblings spent a large part of their early years there as wartime evacuees (they were evacuated to the home of my maternal grandmother!) I was born and wholly brought up in London but was naturally aware of our family background.

Not everyone sees things the same way, I know, but I'm entirely clear of where I stand on the matter of national identity: all nations of the United Kingdom should be proud of their native origin, *as well* as being proud of being British. The fall of Llywelyn ap Gruffudd, the plantations in Ireland, the Act of Union and even the Norman Conquest all happened centuries ago.

In the specific case of Wales, we shouldn't forget that a millennium-and-a-half has gone by since invading Anglo-Saxons drove the Celts west. Since then, most of the families of our nations have intermarried many times. A 'pure' Englishman or Welshman must be a rare, almost non-existent, species. Most of my own family lines were rural Welsh, but I know there are smaller strains of English and Scottish. One of my seventeenth century ancestors was called Elizabeth *Hassan*. This doesn't sound very Welsh or English to me. If I had a narrow nationalist outlook, I'd want to keep a thing like this a secret.

Given the way I see things, my decision to learn Welsh should be no surprise. My attempt in the nineteen-nineties was thwarted by the demands of work. 'Episode One' gave me more time but also difficulty with handling the vital oral side of learning a language. Before the Millennium, I had some degree of competence with French and Spanish, which I had learned in the nineteen-sixties. Still, much of this knowledge had been largely knocked out of my head by what happened to me. How could I even think of trying to improve my frail command of Welsh?

It was 2009 before I had the confidence to try to reach my goal. Although I still then had some verbal difficulties, these were much reduced from what I'd known earlier in the century. So, when I saw the out-of-date advertisement in the shop window, I decided it was time to go for it once again. Imagine my disappointment when 'episode two' forced me to abandon my classes less than a year later.

What should I do now? I didn't want to wait another nine years, even if I could be sure I'd have recovered sufficient of my verbal abilities by then. Welsh is notoriously difficult to pronounce if it's not the speaker's first language. You don't need to think of 'gimmick' words like '*Llanfairpwllgwyngyllgogerychwyrn-drobwllllantysiliogogogoch*' to appreciate this. Try saying more everyday words like 'Llanelli' or 'Chwech' ('six') if you were brought up on the eastern side of the Severn Bridge or north of the River Dee.

You might say it was the very difficulties presented by Welsh pronunciation that came to my aid. My problems with speech made me conscious of the fact that trying to pronounce near tongue-twisters should make an ideal vehicle for the speech exercises I had then started to undertake. The trouble was, I knew it would be highly unfair to expect a teacher and the other students in any evening or day class to endure my laboured efforts. This was when a friend of mine came to my rescue.

I plucked up the courage to ask Joyce to give me one-to-one lessons and, to my huge gratitude, she agreed. She did have some reservations. These weren't about my speech difficulties, but with her own suitability to be a teacher. She'd been brought up speaking Welsh, but these days rarely used it. Furthermore, she had no formal qualifications to teach.

I explained that this would be of no interest to me; I wanted to learn the language for its own sake, not to gain any kind of examination pass. At the personal level, it would be far more important to me if she'd be able to demonstrate patience! At the end of 2011, only a year after my second haemorrhage, we began.

From the outset, I knew I'd been right to count on her patience. Yet she doesn't allow me to get away with carelessness: if my concentration lapses and I pronounce 'y' in the Spanish way or 'un' in the French way, woe betide me. Joyce is never afraid to ask me to repeat things. I'm pleased to note I've been asked to repeat fewer things as time has passed.

A small thing (though not small to me; I'm highly pleased by it) is that when I started to learn I could hardly complete a sentence without a sip from the drink by my side. Now I still have a glass of blackcurrant juice but am pleased to be able to report that I drink more for pleasure than survival these days.

It's not all plain sailing, naturally. The verbal reinforcement so necessary for language learning is necessarily restricted in my case. And, reluctantly, I have to admit that I can't expect to be as sharp-minded as I was in youth. But I do feel I'm going forward. '*En avant!*' Or should I say '*Ymlaen!*'?

## [27] Dreamscapes

When I was younger, I had the most exotic and peculiar dreams. I'm glad to say many of those I have now are still out of the ordinary and often pleasurable. There are, though, a few I'd be happier to do without. These I wish to focus upon here. Someone said the brain uses sleep to unload the debris of life and clear its machinery. I'm inclined to believe this. In the case of the dreams I have noted here they, I'm sure, reflect the anxieties I have at the loss of my former life.

In one I still have fairly frequently, I resumed work after my long absence through illness. Strangely, this was to my old job in Cardiff, not the one in my hometown where I spent the last four years of my employment. Somehow, there existed an understanding that I'd be able to retire through ill health at some undefined time in the near future.

The trouble with my return was that I was far less effective than I'd been before I was unwell. I knew it and the senior management knew it. As a result, I was pushed increasingly further to the margins. This didn't suit my personality, but I no longer had the ability to do much about it.

I found myself doing more and more minor jobs. The worst part of it all was that I knew there was a number of more junior staff who'd be able to make a better job of the various tasks I was undertaking. I tried to ascertain the date when I could leave but couldn't pin this down. At that point I always woke in frustration.

As I've said elsewhere, I don't believe there is really such a thing as 'a sense of direction' but I used to be competent enough at finding my way around. Not so in my dreams, I'm even far worse in those than I am in present-day reality.

In most of the dreams in this category I find myself in a building owned by my former employer in Cardiff. It wasn't where I was working until 1996, though was close to this building and was in a block with which I was perfectly familiar. In fact, I had worked in the offices it housed for about a year in the mid nineteen-seventies. In the dream there is some peculiarity about the lifts between floors.

There actually was some oddity of design, although in reality it was a very minor one. In the dreams, if I didn't take the right turning or get into the appropriate lift it was easy find myself wandering along unfamiliar corridors for what seemed like hours.

Worst of all was the exit from the building. If I came out the wrong way, something easy to do, I'd find myself at its rear. From here, a short walk would take me to unfamiliar parts of the city, miles from where I wanted to be. I'd go on long, circuitous walking routes trying to reach my destination, always the building in which I actually worked up to 1996. In reality this was less than half-a-mile away. It would be almost impossible to lose oneself.

Sometimes my walks around Cardiff would take me to the seafront. This was a wild and desolate shore, nothing like the actuality of what is now called 'Cardiff Bay'. There has been large-scale redevelopment. What was once an industrial area, known simply as 'the docks' or 'Tiger Bay' is now the attractive site of the Wales' Millennium Centre, the Welsh Assembly, plus a host of restaurants and other buildings.

Sometimes, in my anxiety at not being able to find my route I think of getting a taxi. Only then do I discover I have no money. Invariably, I never succeed in finding my way for what in reality is the short distance I want to go before the dreams end, always suddenly and inconclusively.

In a variation of this dream I am on a flight to Australia. For some strange reason, this has a half-hour stopping-off point in South Africa. I've been to Australia and like it a lot but have never been, nor am I likely to go, to South Africa. The dream always takes place at the time of the touchdown to the South African airport.

During the break, to stretch my legs, I take the opportunity to have a walk around the airport. My return to the aeroplane is without incident and made in plenty of time. However, a South African, who has just joined the flight, is sitting in what I assume to be my seat. I remonstrate with him and, quite reasonably and patiently, he shows me his ticket.

This is indeed for the seat he's sitting in. At this point I realise my own place is in the compartment in front of this one. I decide to take the illogical step (as we all know, dreams of any kind rarely follow a logical pattern) of getting off the aeroplane in order to return to the correct compartment.

I disembark, only to discover I can't find any way back onto the aeroplane. I walk all around it, but there doesn't appear to be even a set of gantry steps. Eventually, I do find something, a kind of luggage escalator I remember from a previous airport. Presumably, this was Heathrow. The escalator is not in motion and I know it is not intended for the use passengers: it is cluttered with baggage.

Nevertheless, I decide to ascend. With difficulty, I clamber upwards, only to decide half-way up that the suitcases and bags are providing too much of an obstacle. I then realise the conveyor wouldn't have taken me where I wanted to go, anyway. At this point I look at my wristwatch and see that it is 1:15pm. This is the scheduled time for the flight to resume. At this point I wake up, although the real hour is half-way through the night, rather than in the early afternoon.

Fortunately, most of my dreams still provide good experiences. When I was young this was especially so. I know I was not alone in regularly dreaming I had the ability to fly and accepted this as entirely normal. I still have such dreams, though more often these days I am restricted to a kind of 'long-hopping' or floating above the ground. It's still a satisfying experience, though perhaps this is an indication that I'm getting older and more responsible!

One dream I occasionally experience combines the old and the new in a strange and not altogether happy way. In this, I start off by 'long-hopping' but soon ascend higher. I find myself thinking 'Good. I can fly properly again.' I glide around, finding myself in an unwelcome landscape of grey-brown mounds.

I decide these are formed by the industrial mining of clay, even though the quarry mounds are far higher than any that would be the by-product of a real-life clay-pit extraction. I want to fly away from this bleak landscape to find somewhere more interesting, but discover the workings cover a wide area and I can't find my way out of it. For some reason, although they don't play an important part in the mechanics of the process, my shoulders start to ache through all the flying.

They are still aching when I wake up.

## [28] Writing

A few years ago, I wrote a piece for my friend Sam Kates' blog. I called it *Why Write*. This is part of it:

*'Leaving aside more mundane demands like shopping lists and business writing, plus shorter things like personal emails (not to say some of these* shouldn't *be creative) it seemed to me there are three main reasons to write. In* reverse *order of importance, I have always considered these to be:*

1.     *To make money.*
2.     *To express your thoughts to others.*
3.     *Because that demon keeps jab-jab-jabbing away at us and* making *us write.*

*N years after I first wrote for publication, this is still the way I see things. I have, though, recently modified my view to an extent.*

*When I lived in London, back in the Dark Ages (well, it was a long time ago) I wrote a few things commercially or semi-commercially. This first period of literary activity lasted for not much more than two years before 'life got in the way' and my attention went in other directions. This period of comparative dormancy went on for a number of years. I* did *do some creative writing in this interval – I didn't seem to have any choice in the matter – but didn't try to get anything published.*

*Then, following a trip to Romania in 1988, at the time when Nicolae Ceauşescu was still dictator, I was bursting with ideas I had to express, in prose and poetry, in fiction and non-fiction. At that time, the outlet most readily available was the small press, so this was where I initially concentrated my efforts.*

*The first thing I wrote (an essay; nothing to do with Romania as it happens) appeared in* Schools Poetry Review *in 1989. After this, over the years, I have published around 200 poems, about 80 short stories and roughly the same number of commercial features. Added to this is a large number of works of reviews, essays and things I can best describe as 'other prose'.*

*I also wrote six (print) books of various kinds.*

*Given what I said earlier about motives for writing, you'd think I should have been happy. If I hadn't made enormous sums of money, I do know that a largish number of people have read what I've had to say and at least I've managed to keep that demon and his pitchfork still. There were, though, two large flies in the ointment. Firstly, much of my writing had to be undertaken against the background of a busy and demanding job. Secondly, several years ago life got in the way again, more negatively this time, just when my literary life was showing signs of taking off.'*

This book has gone into some detail about the way 'life got in the way again' for me.

Months after I came out of hospital in the Millennium year, I felt impelled to make some money by writing commercial features. This wasn't through financial necessity but because of a psychological need to gain some earned income again. I quite enjoyed much of what I did and was reasonably successful at it. However, it slowly dawned on me that, unless you're a 'name' writer, the hourly rate for writing commercial features is poor.

Gradually I came to write fewer magazine articles and these days I write more of the things I want to express. Some of my recent efforts are listed at the back of this volume. You could say my number one priority has become once again to silence that demon with his pitchfork.

## [29] Quo Vadis?

Where am I going?

Well, I certainly don't think I'm some kind of latter-day St Peter, that's for sure. My intention is to keep up my daily speech practice, maintain reasonable fitness and activity, watch my intake of food and drink, try to keep my mind alert and to maintain an interest in the world about me for as long as I can.

In other words, apart from the first, to continue to try to do all things we should all be trying to do.

Of course, I recognise the years are slipping by. I'm lucky in that I think I let them slip by fairly easily, even now. I've had my turn at being young and I enjoyed it. Where am I going? Where is any one of us going?

A peculiar but pleasant sensation I found early in the century was that of feeling younger as time passed. This feeling was the direct result of my recovery progressing. It was of course illusory because my illness caused the clock to be turned forward in the first place. Only then could I enjoy the benefits of feeling the clock ticking backwards. Nevertheless, this sensation lasted right up until the time that 'episode two' arrived to wind my life forward once again, though I don't believe this was for too long.

I have to acknowledge that the years are passing and I can't expect to have the illusion of cheating the clock for ever – not that I'd want it to if part of the deal was a health drama every ten years! Still, it does gives me pleasure now to be able to do small things like walking down the steps from my local rugby club stand more easily than I could even a year or two ago.

Octogenarians and Nonagenarians who respond to the gift of life in a positive way are people I admire greatly. I know several people who have reached or surpassed this exalted level of seniority but am going confine myself to just two examples.

The first was someone I originally knew in the nineteen-seventies. Ted was a former local politician and I knew him first of all in a work environment. The circumstances of our re-acquaintance in early 2006 were different.

I was researching a feature I was writing on Kenfig. This was known as the 'City Under the Sands' because the medieval settlement and twelfth century castle had been engulfed by sand dunes, leaving rich material for historians.

One aspect I wanted to cover in the feature was the legal dispute between the ancient corporation of Kenfig and the then British Steel Company. This ran from 1959 to 1971 and ended in the High Court. I remember the question I asked a friend: 'Who is the Man of Kenfig?' The answer came back unhesitatingly 'Ted'.

This pleased me no end. Through his son, Derek, whom I knew independently, Suki and I arranged to go to see him. We received the warmest of welcomes. Ted, who by then was then 93, made us a cup of tea and gave us a slice of cake he'd made himself. He was able to answer my many questions and found some excellent photographs I was pleased to use with the article.

His account of the Borough's legal dispute about water supply with British Steel was sharp and complete. This could have ended in the week before; not nearly 35 years previously, such was the vivacity of what he told us. Ted was Chairman of the ancient Borough in 1971. He was still the Chairman in 2006.

I well remember him telling me of officials coming around to value his house. He'd have been personally liable if the court case had been lost. As it was, the Borough won. The corporation could prove title to the 90-acre Kenfig Pool and other land and property surrounding it. The main purpose of their meetings now is to award bursaries from the funds generated by their property. So, the shifting sands of Kenfig finally did the local population some good.

Ted still drove and he told us that the cake he'd given us had been baked by him at a local evening class he was attending. Cookery wouldn't have been his first choice of evening study, but it was all that was available locally. I complimented him on the way he was keeping himself active. He said to me:

'Tom, the day I stop wanting to do things is the day they can come around to measure me up for a wooden overcoat'. He laughed as he said this. I joined in his laughter, considering myself privileged to be able to do so. I can quote his words exactly because Suki noted them down when he spoke them.

The other person I want to mention is Wes. He is a highly active man, attending many events within a range of thirty or forty miles to read poetry. The thing that most sticks in my mind, though, has nothing to do with the reading of poetry. In response to a casual question of mine, he told me that he and his wife Linda had been for a longish walk on Boxing Day, 2015. Both were then in their mid-eighties and I commended Wes on his enterprise. He said:

'We're always being told we should take more exercise. It's when we're older we need it more.' Indeed.

The last two years have not been easy for me. About four years ago, I was diagnosed with glaucoma in one eye. But the diagnosis was made at an early stage and the condition is controlled by a single eye drop daily. I'm hopeful that this will be the case for many years to come.

But then, a few years later came Suki's illness and passing. This was my hardest time, harder than any part of my life, either before or since. Suki was the love of my life. Many people have done their best to help me through and I am so grateful for this.

Only a few months afterwards and as we all know, the virus (SARS-CoV-2, to give its full ugly name) came upon the World. We may not yet – I write this in the summer of 2020 – have seen the worst of the pandemic's depredations. I also personally believe that the social damage, including the economic damage, could be more harmful in the long term than the effect upon global health. Even so, you'll understand if I see the pandemic, in comparison to what happened before, as something of a bump in the road.

But we'll all do our best to get through these things, won't we?

# Appendices

## APPENDIX 1: Diary of events, put together with help from Suki, in second half of April, 2000

21st March – 22nd March, 2000 Casualty Unit 9:30pm – 1:30am

- Smiling at Suki. She stayed overnight 21st-23rd and 26th until discharge. Joseph also stayed on night of 21st
- Trying to obey doctor but unable to respond by lifting right foot, leg or hand, also speech very bad
- Chest X-ray
- Computerised tomography scan of brain (deeper scan than X-ray, would show actual site of bleeding)
- Reports from CT scan to Casualty
- 1:30am Medical Assessment Unit transfer

22nd March, 2000 Medical Assessment Unit

- Six staff necessary to hold me down to fit 'main line' for hydration and administration of drugs to control blood pressure.
- Late AM, moved to Ward 4

24th March, 2000 Ward 4
- Hydration only until this stage
- Assessment of swallowing reflex made
- Dr Helen Parry came to administer 'Isoket' to control blood pressure
- Edmund stayed overnight

25th March, 2000
- First breakfast
- Joseph stayed overnight

26th March, 2000 - 30th March, 2000
- Visitors were stopped because I was becoming agitated.

28th March, 2000
- Moved to side ward and stayed there until discharge

29th March, 2000
- Isoket stopped; blood pressure OK.

30th March, 2000
- Physiotherapist (Siân) came to teach exercises to do in bed.

31st March, 2000
- Sat up for meals

1st April, 2000
- Walked in room

2nd April, 2000
- Walked in ward with boys. I have more or less continuous memories from this date.

11th March, 2000
- Discharged. Breda gave us lift home.

# APPENDIX 2 – Notes and Drawings Made on 9th April, 2000

| DATE | CLINICAL NOTES (Each entry must be signed) |
|---|---|
| 1 | THOUGHT HEAVENS |
| 2 | HEAEN WARS                9/4/2000 |
| 3 | BLUE HEAVEN |
| 4 | BEN |
| 4 | BEING A NUISANSE |
| 5 | |
| 6 | |
| 7 | |
| 8 | WHO'S THAT DOWN SAFE A THERAPIST! |

# APPENDIX 3 – Notes Made on 10th April, 2000

| CONTINUATION HISTORY SHEET | SURNAME Mr/Mrs/Miss FIRST NAMES | CASE No. |
|---|---|---|

| DATE | CLINICAL NOTES (Each entry must be signed) |
|---|---|
| 10/04/2000 | |

Monday

I'm bored!

I May write like a "nichot"
But I'm not one!

I'm gently mobile

This is. the each and every end ─ ─ ─ .

## APPENDIX 4: 'Script' for telephone call 11th February, 2011

Hello Stephanie. It's Tom. We'll be seeing you tomorrow.

We hope you had a good week off.

Can you do me a favour please? It's not urgent; it can wait until 21st. I've lost one of my magic laminated cards, so would you mind doing me another?

The wording is, 'I have a speech difficulty, but I can understand.'

Again: 'I have a speech difficulty, but I can understand'.

Thanks.

## APPENDIX 5: Letter to a Well-Wisher, August, 2000

Thank you for your letter of 23 June, 2000, and my apologies for the belated reply.

Unfortunately, the incident was of fairly serious proportions, but I am pleased to say that I am making a very good recovery. One of the residual problems means that I can't type as quickly as I could and write by hand even more slowly (that's my excuse for not replying earlier). Perhaps the best thing I can do is quote from a letter to our holiday insurers. It's a bit clinical but you'll get the drift.

*'Prior to the incident I enjoyed very good health. The only effects which I suffer now are to my vision, where I can see double on occasion; my speech, where I suffer a slight impediment; and to my manual dexterity on my right-side where I am not as quick as I was. These residual problems continue to improve. On the plus side I have retained all my faculties, and my mobility is excellent - I regularly walk the mile-and-a-half to town and on two occasions I have walked 4-5 miles without difficulty. I have responded to the medication, which in both cases is intended to control my blood pressure. This is now consistently about 125/80 (that's good). The medication I take is 50mg Atenolol and 5mg Amlodipine, neither of which have any discernible side effects. In both cases the dosage has been halved from that originally prescribed. I do not have any special needs at all on my holiday.'*

Thanks too for your story, which I haven't yet discussed with Arthur. I have had a host of well-wishers, by telephone, in writing, and via personal visit. It looks as if I'll have to give up work, which is about three years early for me with my sons either at or about to go to University. But *c'est la vie* and taking everything into account I was extremely lucky. Your husband will be green with envy (or has he managed to finish yet?)

Could I put right a misconception? I know the timing is rather frightening, but I'd decided to drop the *Review*, and discussed it with Arthur, before I had the stroke. The reasons, apart from the ones I gave in the magazine (which I stand by) are that the exercise was a little time consuming, and I wanted to increase the time I had available for paid work.

I've had to review my decision in the light of my stroke, but it still holds good, even though I'll have more time for writing in the future. At present my slowness in typing has meant that I've entered the business of full-time writing slowly and have taken up just a few paid commissions.

But I'm improving almost daily now. Within a month or two I'll genuinely be a full-time writer. So there!

All the best and thanks for your support.

## APPENDIX 6: Speech Therapy, Part One (Poem)

### Speech Therapy Part 1
#### I

**It started like this:**

> This is a strong, silent, poem.
> **[Pause].**
> At least it's silent.
> **[Pause].**
> And there are lots of pauses.
> **[Pause].**
>
> 'Slow down,' she says.
> **[Pause].**
> But if I slow down any more.
> **[Pause].**
> I'll come to a complete stop.
> **[Pause].**
>
> Sorry, this is the best I can do at the moment.
> **[Pause].**
> That was a long line.
> But I'll be
> **[Pause]**
> back.

#### II

**I had a speech therapist.**

> Stephanie knew her stuff.
> But the six weeks went.
> She was a speech therapist, not the sugar-plum fairy.
> She said, 'Give yourself formal therapy sessions.
> You've got the tool kit.'

## III

**It was thirty months before I could cope.**

I tried poetry:
> '*I met a traveller from antique land*
> *Who said: "Two vast and trunkless legs of stone*
> *Stand in the desert. Near them on the sand…'*

> '*…only awoke paint-box images*
> *of steep streets and hills at the end of a cloud:*
> *slate-grey, misty green, and always wet…'*

Stair-counting:
> '*Ein, zwei, drei…*
> *Satu, dua, tiga…*
> *Un, doi, trei…'*

Even singing:
> '*Frankie and Johnnie were lovers*
> *O Lordie how they could love…'*

It's a long road.
But I'll be back.

***Chris says:*** 'I had an idea for a poem for you to write. It would be called *Speech Therapy* (oh yes it would!). It would have 2 parts. The first part would be an attempt at writing a poem that would sound like you now. I'd imagine it would be heavily vowel-based and be d-r-a-w-n-o-u-t and meant to be read slowly. The second part would be something to aim at reading out in a couple of months, which would be faster, more consonant-based and staccato.'

***I say:*** 'Surely you didn't expect me to obey *rules*? But *Speech Therapy Part One* is the nearest I'm going to get for a while. Don't expect *Speech Therapy Part Two* in the next few months!'

## APPENDIX 7: Speech Therapy, Part Two (Poem)

### Speech Therapy Part Two
*[I hope not 2 of 999]*

And so, I plod my twelve steps;
up the stairs. Down the stairs.
*Un, dau, tri.*
*Un, deux, trois.*
*Uno, dos, tres.*
I'm running low on language ease.
I'll have to awaken my flaky Cantonese
*Yāt, Yih, Sàam*
or learn to count past ten in Breton
*unan, daou, tri,*
*pevar, pemp, c'hwec'h, seizh, eizh, nav, dek.*
Oh, all right then: *unnek, daouzek.*


But I know the difference between **_gau_** and **gau**.
(Did you hear it just now?
I didn't know I could be so deft.
If you didn't blush, you're just tone deaf).


I took my exercises Down Under.
It was good to sing under the southern sun
with Tyson the German Shepherd looking on in wonder:
*Frankie and Johnnie were lovers,*
*O Lordie, how they could love....*
The views of neighbour Serge might have been other.


Unwisely, I sometimes go for
trying to talk over
the rubbish music at the rugby.
I can't do this.
But then, neither can Chris.

I joked that by the time I was one hundred and sixty-three
I'd be word perfect and free.
Then it became one hundred and sixty-four.
then one hundred and sixty-five.
Now the joke sounds contrived.

But at least when I say the name 'Boris Johnson'
(I like a bit of satire)
people now understand what I mean.

Or at least I'm older and wiser.

## APPENDIX 8: The Speech Cards

**The Original, From February, 2011**

I have a speech difficulty

but I can understand

**The Copy Made in Malaysia**

I have a speech difficulty

but I can understand

## APPENDIX 9: Activities During Ambulatory Blood Pressure Monitoring.

28th February, 2011

| | |
|---|---|
| 12:00 | Return home from hospital via bus. |
| 12:30 | Taking coat off |
| 13:00 | Eating lunch |
| 13:30 | Working on computer |
| 14:45 | Read |
| 15:05 | Sleep |
| 15:25 | Read |
| 16:00 | Watch TV |
| 17:05 | Miscellaneous Activities |
| 18:00 | Watch TV |
| 18:35 | Shave |
| 18:50 | Miscellaneous Activities |
| 19:30 | Watch TV |
| 22:15 | Bed (sleep approx. 22:35) |

1st March 2011

| | |
|---|---|
| 03:00 | Awoken by monitor activity |
| 03:45 | Sleep |
| 04:00 | Awoken by monitor activity |
| 06:15 | Sleep |
| 07:50 | Awake |
| 08:30 | Dressing |
| 09:00 | Breakfast |
| 09:20 | Turned monitor off |

## Recently by Tom East

### *NOVELS*
***The Gospel According to St Judas***
***The Greenland Party***
***Tommy's War: July, 1914***

### *THE ELDRITCH COLLECTIONS*
***The Eve of St Eligius***
***Wish Man's Wood***

### *OTHER FICTION*
***Dimension Five***

### *NON-FICTION*
***A Fifties Childhood***

### *POETRY*
***Scenes from Seasons***
***Charge of The Light Verse Brigade***
***Lyrics, Polemics & Poetics***

Coming next,
more non-fiction:
*Why Write Haiku?*

Printed in Great Britain
by Amazon

14631191R00092